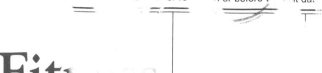

Fit...

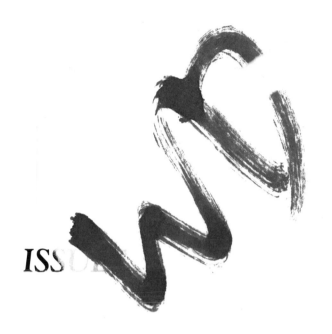

ISS...

Volume 61

Editor

Craig Donnellan

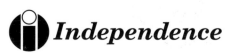

Independence

Educational Publishers
Cambridge

First published by Independence
PO Box 295
Cambridge CB1 3XP
England

© Craig Donnellan 2003

British Library Cataloguing in Publication Data
Fitness – (Issues Series)
I. Donnellan, Craig II. Series
613.7

ISBN 1 86168 231 X

Printed in Great Britain
MWL Print Group Ltd

Typeset by
Claire Boyd

Cover
The illustration on the front cover is by
Pumpkin House.

CONTENTS

Chapter One: How Fit Are We?

Chapter Two: Physical Exercise

Introduction

Fitness is the sixty-first volume in the **Issues** series. The aim of this series is to offer up-to-date information about important issues in our world.

Fitness examines how fit we are, our diets and the benefits of a healthy diet and an active lifestyle.

The information comes from a wide variety of sources and includes:
Government reports and statistics
Newspaper reports and features
Magazine articles and surveys
Web site material
Literature from lobby groups
and charitable organisations.

It is hoped that, as you read about the many aspects of the issues explored in this book, you will critically evaluate the information presented. It is important that you decide whether you are being presented with facts or opinions. Does the writer give a biased or an unbiased report? If an opinion is being expressed, do you agree with the writer?

Fitness offers a useful starting-point for those who need convenient access to information about the many issues involved. However, it is only a starting-point. At the back of the book is a list of organisations which you may want to contact for further information.

*****

Overweight pupils 'doing hardly any exercise'

For many, daily activity is just walking to and from classrooms, say experts

By Suzanne Finney

Many schoolchildren do as little as 24 minutes of 'moderate' exercise a day, according to a study.

Such activity can include walking to and from classrooms or climbing stairs.

In contrast, the British Heart Foundation recommends 30 minutes of 'proper' exercise five times a week – including swimming, netball, football, tennis and rounders.

The report comes only days after it emerged that parents could soon start outliving their offspring because of an obesity epidemic among youngsters.

Experts at Bristol University, who are monitoring activity rates among overweight children aged from four to 18, found that only five per cent of youngsters walk or cycle to school. Twenty years ago, the figure was 80 per cent.

And more than 30 per cent of the children studied by a team led by Dr Angie Page showed low levels of activity, with teenage girls doing the least.

Overall, older children appeared to engage in less exercise than younger pupils.

Dr Page, a lecturer at the university, said: 'We found some were doing less than one or two minutes of moderate activity an hour, which is a lower figure than we've seen from other data.

'Teenage girls tended to do less than teenage boys and the older children did less than the younger ones.'

She will deliver her findings to an Association for the Study of Obesity conference in Bristol this week. The scaling down of sport in schools and the continued selling off of playing fields have been widely blamed for the drastic decline in exercise.

Meanwhile, an EU meeting on obesity in Copenhagen last week heard that Britain has the fastest growing obesity rate in Europe.

Youngsters' fat-laden diets and their lack of exercise has resulted in a record number of them being so grossly overweight that they run the

Ten per cent of children starting primary school are now regarded as alarmingly overweight

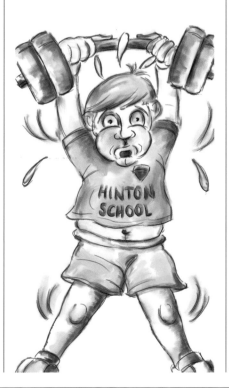

risk of early death due to diabetes, heart attack of stroke.

Experts warned that many such teenagers also risk going blind or needing kidney transplants as a result of diabetes in their 30s, which would place huge demands on the health service. They urged the Government to force the fast-food industry to carry health food warnings on high-fat foods in the same way the tobacco industry places health warnings on cigarette packets.

Ten per cent of children starting primary school are now regarded as alarmingly overweight, increasing to 15 per cent among school leavers.

Doctors fear this could lead to three out of four Britons being labelled obese within the next 15 years.

Medics believe the condition is likely to overtake smoking as the country's number one preventable killer.

Dr Julian Shield, a senior lecturer in metabolics at Bristol University, has diagnosed early onset Type 2 diabetes in eight young patients.

He said: 'Children with a weight problem are all too aware society doesn't view them favourably.

'As they get fat they become more reclusive, go out less and do less exercise.'

Type 2 diabetes is almost exclusively triggered by being overweight and a diet high in sugar and fat.

David Barker, of the British Heart Foundation, said: 'Young people can keep a healthy heart by eating fresh fruit and vegetables and making sure they get 30 minutes of exercise a day, five times a week.'

© *The Daily Mail*
September 2002

Plucky pensioners outpace teens

New research by Dr Kimberly Fisher of the Institute for Social and Economic Research (ISER) reveals that the average young person in Britain spends less time engaged in physical activity than the average pensioner.

On the average day, people aged between 8 and 19 spend 1 hour and 15 minutes doing any form of physical activity, while those aged over 65 tend to be active for 1 hour and 40 minutes. The gap is large enough to reflect a real difference in lifestyle between younger and older people. And the sedentary lifestyle of the younger generation has potentially damaging consequences for their future health.

Dr Fisher has examined data from the National Survey of Time Use, which was conducted by the Office for National Statistics and released earlier this year. This study is based on a random national sample of around 5,000 households. All people aged 8 and older in these households were asked to keep a diary of their activities over two randomly selected days, one weekday and one weekend day.

The study examined time spent in a range of physical activities: sports and exercise; walking dogs; physically active housework, such as vacuuming, moving furniture and many forms of DIY; productive exercise, such as turning soil in an allotment by hand or picking berries; and travel on foot or bicycle. Dr Fisher's analysis of the responses reveals that:

- Young people are more active on days when they are not in school, but even on these days, teenage boys are only as active as older men, and teenage girls are still less active than older women.
- On any given day, nearly 20% of Britons do no physical activity that lasts longer than 5 consecutive minutes. While only 12% of people aged 65+ are this inactive, 22% of people aged 8-35 did no exercise lasting at least 10 minutes in their day.
- Though boys are more physically active than girls, after the age of 20, women tend to be more physically active than men. At all ages, men spend more time than women playing sports, but women spend more time than men walking, cycling and doing physically active housework as adults.
- Diarists were asked if they had participated in any of 43 sports in the last four weeks. Over half said they played some sports on at least a monthly basis. But at the same time, approaching half of the sample – 42% (4,229 people) – indicated that they had not participated in any sport – not even keep-fit exercises – over the last four weeks.
- People who say they almost always feel rushed are less likely to participate in sports and keep-fit exercise during a month than people who only occasionally feel rushed. Yet people who seldom or never feel time pressured are even less likely than those who always feel rushed to participate in sports.
- More curiously, people who have access to the internet at home are more likely to participate in sports than those who do not have internet access at home. This association holds across the age groups, and is particularly large for people in the older working age groups.

On any given day, nearly 20% of Britons do no physical activity that lasts longer than 5 consecutive minutes

---

The diary data only show the time in which people are active, not the intensity of exercise or the number of calories people burn while doing exercise. Even so, young people naturally have more potential energy to spend than pensioners. People's lifestyle choices in youth can significantly influence their chances of health in older age. Young people who lead a sedentary lifestyle face greater risks of obesity and health problems in later life.

Note

Chewing the fat – the story time diaries tell about physical activity in the United Kingdom by Kimberly Fisher will be published – 2 September 2002 – by the Institute for Social and Economic Research (ISER) at the University of Essex as ISER Working Paper 2002-13.

- The above information is from the Institute for Social and Economic Research's (ISER) web site which can be found at www.iser.essex.ac.uk

Physical activity and youth

Information from the World Health Organization (WHO)

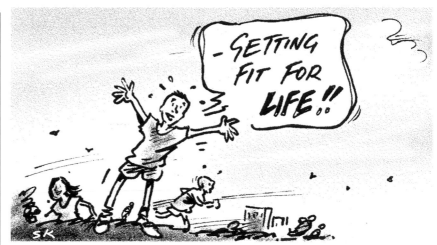

Regular physical activity provides young people with important physical, mental and social health benefits. Regular practice of physical activity helps children and young people to build and maintain healthy bones, muscles and joints, helps control body weight, helps reduce fat and develop efficient function of the heart and lungs. It contributes to the development of movement and co-ordination and helps prevent and control feelings of anxiety and depression.

Play, games and other physical activities give young people opportunities for self-expression, building self-confidence, feelings of achievement, social interaction and integration. These positive effects also help counteract the risks and harm caused by the demanding, competitive, stressful and sedentary way of life that is so common in young people's lives today. Involvement in properly guided physical activity and sports can also foster the adoption of other healthy behaviour including avoidance of tobacco, alcohol and drug use and violent behaviour. It can also foster healthy diet, adequate rest and better safety practices.

Some studies show that among adolescents, the more often they participate in physical activity, the less likely they are to use tobacco. It has also been found that children who are more physically active showed higher academic performance. Team games and play promote positive social integration and facilitate the development of social skills in young children.

Patterns of physical activity acquired during childhood and adolescence are more likely to be maintained throughout the life span, thus providing the basis for active and healthy life. On the other hand, unhealthy lifestyles – including sedentary lifestyle, poor diet and substance abuse – adopted at a young age are likely to persist in adulthood.

Physical activity levels are decreasing among young people in countries around the world, especially in poor urban areas. It is estimated that less than one-third of young people are sufficiently active to benefit their present and future health and well-being.

Physical education and other school-based physical activities are also decreasing. Only a few countries offer at least two hours per week of physical education in both primary and secondary schools. These negative trends are likely to continue, even worsen and spread to an increasing number of countries.

This decline is largely due to increasingly common sedentary ways of life. For example fewer children walk or cycle to school and excessive time is devoted to watching television, playing computer games, and using computers – very often at the expense of time and opportunities for physical activity and sports.

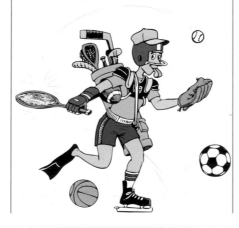

Many factors prevent young people from being regularly physically active: lack of time and motivation, insufficient support and guidance from adults, feelings of embarrassment or incompetence, lack of safe facilities and locales for physical activity, and simple ignorance of the benefits of physical activity.

Schools present unique opportunities to provide time, facilities and guidance for physical activity for young people. Schools have the mandate and responsibility for enhancing all aspects of growth and development for children and young people. In most countries, through physical education programmes, schools offer the only systematic opportunity for young people to take part in and learn about physical activity.

Ample participation in play, games and other physical activities, both in school and during free time, is essential for the healthy development of every young person. Access to safe places, opportunities and time, and good examples from teachers, parents and friends are all part of ensuring that children and young people move for health.

■ The above information is from World Health Organization's web site which can be found at www.who.int

© 2002 WHO/OMS

Physical activity and coronary heart disease

People who are physically active have a lower risk of coronary heart disease (CHD). To produce the maximum benefit the activity needs to be regular and aerobic. Aerobic activity involves using the large muscle groups in the arms, legs and back steadily and rhythmically so that breathing and heart rate are significantly increased.

It is estimated that about 36% of deaths from CHD in men and 38% of deaths from CHD in women are due to lack of physical activity and that 9% of deaths from CHD in the UK could be avoided if people who are currently sedentary or have a light level of physical activity increased their level of physical activity to a moderate level.[1]

The Government recommendation on physical activity is that adults should participate in a minimum of 30 minutes of at least moderate intensity activity (such as brisk walking, cycling or climbing the stairs) on five or more days of the week.[2,3]

Overall levels of physical activity

Physical activity levels are low in the UK: only 37% of men and 25% of women meet the current guidelines (30 minutes' moderate activity on five or more days a week) suggested by the Government. In addition, over one-third of adults are currently inactive, that is do less than one occasion of 30 minutes' activity a week.

Age and sex differences

Physical activity declines rapidly with age. Whereas 58% of men and 33% of women aged 16-24 are physically active for 30 minutes or more at least five days a week, this declines to 17% of men and 12% of women in the 65-74 age group.

It is recommended that all children and young people aged 5-18 participate in physical activity of at least moderate intensity for one hour a day.[4] In England, 55% of boys aged 2-15 and 39% of girls, are active for at least an hour on five or more days a week. Participation rates decline with age after around 8-10 years, with the decline steepest in girls. By the age of 15, only 18% of girls reach the recommended level of activity.

Temporal trends

It is generally thought that over the last 20 years physical activity levels have declined in the UK.[5] Since 1994 the proportion meeting the current recommended level of physical activity has remained stable at 37% in men and increased slightly, from 22% to 25% in women; but the

---

It is estimated that about 36% of deaths from CHD in men and 38% of deaths from CHD in women are due to lack of physical activity

---

proportion classified as sedentary (less than one occasion of physical activity of thirty minutes a week) has increased from 30% in 1994 to 35% in 1998 in men, and from 35% to 41% in women.

Socio-economic differences

Socio-economic differences in physical activity are complex. In men, overall activity levels are greater in manual social classes than in non-manual classes: half of those working in unskilled manual employment meet current recommended levels compared to just under a third of those in professional jobs. In women, however, there is no clear pattern according to social class in the proportion meeting the recommended activity level.

The type of activity, however, does vary with social class in men and women, with more work-related activity in manual (especially in men) and sports activity (especially in women) in non-manual classes.[6]

Overall activity levels vary by household income in men, being highest among those with mid-range

Premature deaths from circulatory diseases

The United Kingdom has one of the highest premature death rates from circulatory disease (which includes heart disease and stroke) in Europe, after the Irish Republic and Finland. For those aged under 65, the rate for the United Kingdom in 1998 was almost twice the rate in France, the country with the lowest death rate. A number of risk factors known to increase a person's risk of circulatory disease have been identified, included drinking alcohol, smoking, obesity and the lack of regular exercise.

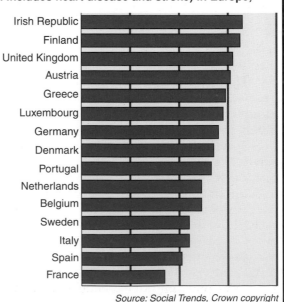

Irish Republic
Finland
United Kingdom
Austria
Greece
Luxembourg
Germany
Denmark
Portugal
Netherlands
Belgium
Sweden
Italy
Spain
France

Source: Social Trends, Crown copyright

household incomes and lowest at both extremes of the income distribution. No pattern is apparent in women. However, participation in two specific types of physical activity, sports/exercise and walking, increases with income in both men and women.[7]

Ethnic differences

Compared with the general population, South Asian and Chinese men and women are less likely to participate in physical activity, with the lowest levels found in the Bangladeshi community. Only 18% of Bangladeshi men and 7% of Bangladeshi women meet the current recommended physical activity levels (30 minutes' activity on five or more days a week). African Caribbean men and women are the most likely to be physically active at the recommended level.

International differences

Levels of activity vary across European member states, with levels of activity in the UK falling below the EU average.

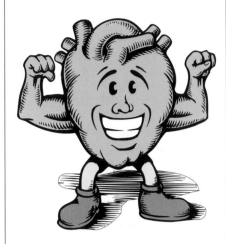

Public health targets

Only Scotland and Northern Ireland have physical activity targets.

Sources:

1. National Heart Forum. *Coronary heart disease: Estimating the impact of changes in risk factors.* The Stationery Office: London (in press).
2. Department of Health (1996) *Strategy Statement of Physical Activity.* DH: London.
3. It should be noted that the recommended activity levels for Northern Ireland and Scotland are age-related and combine the guidelines on vigorous and moderate intensity activity.
4. Biddle S, Sallis J and Cavill N (eds). (1998) *Young and Active? Young people and health enhancing physical activity – evidence and implications.* Health Education Authority: London.
5. Prentice AM, Jebb SA (1995) Obesity in Britain: gluttony or sloth? *British Medical Journal* 311: 437-9.
6. See Figure 5.14 p211, Joint Health Surveys Unit (1999) *Health Survey for England 1998.* The Stationery Office: London.
7. See Figure 5I, p193, Joint Health Surveys Unit (1999) *Health Survey for England 1998.* The Stationery Office: London.

■ The above information is an extract from Coronary Heart Statistics produced by the British Heart Foundation. See page 41 for their address details.

Obesity linked to TVs in toddlers' bedrooms

By Martin Wainwright

Almost 10 years after the triumphant birth of the children's TV programme *Teletubbies*, scientists have proved that the fat little creatures exist in real life.

The first research into TV and pre-school obesity has nailed under-fours' increasingly common girdle of unwanted fat firmly on the growing practice of giving toddlers their own bedroom TVs.

Almost 3,000 roly-polys aged under five were interviewed in the United States, where the 'square-eyed babysitter' is an increasingly popular way of keeping small children quiet. Comparative studies were made with obese teenagers and adults, whose weight gain has already been linked to couch potatodom.

The study by Columbia University and a New York healthcare institute found that 40% of the children – including all the chubbiest – already had their own bedroom TVs. Overall, they heavily outweighed the rest of the sample who did not have a bedroom set.

The study warns that peer pressure is certain to increase the problem, which is likely to affect Europe too. The survey also found that, like the Jesuits, a bedroom TV which gets a child before five, wins allegiance for life.

Viewing by the bedroom sample as they got older increased significantly faster than among the rest of the children monitored by the researchers.

The report, published today in the *American Journal of Paediatrics*, concludes: 'A TV in the child's bedroom is the strongest marker of increased risk of being overweight. Because most children watch TV by age two, educational efforts about limiting child TV/video viewing and keeping the TV out of the child's bedroom need to begin before then.'

Obese children

How overweight children of five are showing early signs of heart disease

By Beezy Marsh,
Medical Reporter

Obese children as young as five are displaying signs of heart disease, doctors warned yesterday.

Nearly 60 per cent of seriously overweight youngsters aged five to ten have at least one symptom which raises the risk of the illness that leads to heart attacks.

Some obese children have 'clusters' of symptoms, including high blood pressure, raised levels of blood fats, which can clog arteries, and changes in insulin levels.

Some youngsters also have an increased risk of asthma, breathing difficulties and joint and liver problems.

The shocking findings, which emerged at the UK's first major conference on childhood obesity in Bristol, follow warnings last week from medical experts that the parents of today may outlive their obese children.

The conference was told that childhood obesity has reached epidemic proportions.

Rates of serious weight problems have risen dramatically over the past decade, with nearly a third of children aged 16 classified overweight, and 17 per cent of 15-year-olds obese.

The trend is affecting even the very young, with around one in ten six-year-olds classed as obese and more than one in five overweight.

Girls are marginally more likely to have weight problems than boys. Couch-potato lifestyles coupled with a diet rich in fat and sugar are largely to blame.

Despite the trend, parents, teachers and even some doctors fail to see childhood obesity as a health problem. Some believe the child will simply grow out of it.

> *Girls are marginally more likely to have weight problems than boys. Couch-potato lifestyles coupled with a diet rich in fat and sugar are largely to blame*

Nutritionists at Glasgow University carried out a review of research in 39 medical journals to reveal the threat to children's health.

Dr John Reilly, of the university's Department of Human Nutrition, told the Association for the Study of Obesity yesterday: 'There is a fairly common perception among families or health professionals that it doesn't matter that much if a child is overweight – it is purely a cosmetic problem.

'In fact, there are some strong associations between obesity in childhood and future consequences for health.'

Among the most alarming findings were that in obese boys and girls aged five to ten, 58 per cent showed early signs of heart disease. Levels of 'bad' fats, which lead to clogging of arteries in middle age, are already rising due to their weight.

Coronary heart disease afflicts around two million Britons and claims the life of one person every three minutes – making it Britain's biggest killer. Overweight children are also showing signs of insulin changes – which could be linked to diabetes.

A study from the Royal Hospital for Sick Children in Bristol last year found signs of Type Two diabetes, which is linked to being overweight, in obese children as young as 13.

High blood pressure in childhood could also lead to an increased risk of strokes.

Dr Reilly said of the obesity epidemic: 'All the signs suggest it is going to get worse before it gets better.'

Belinda Linden, cardiac care nurse at the British Heart Foundation, said the charity was very concerned about the rising tide of childhood obesity.

'Our biggest concern is that we are going to see more people in middle age suffering an illness,' she said.

'The difficulty is trying to get children to understand that what they eat and do today may have a bearing on their health tomorrow. Tomorrow is a long time for a child.'

© *The Daily Mail*
September 2002

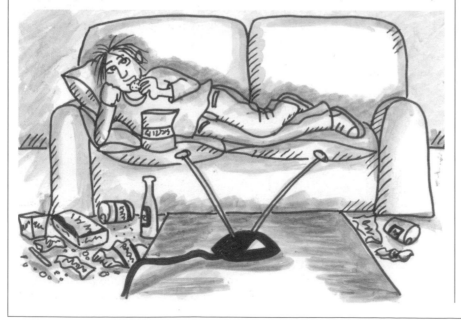

Hungry for change

Multinationals, ready meals and malnutrition – why fat is a socialist issue

By Jeanette Winterson

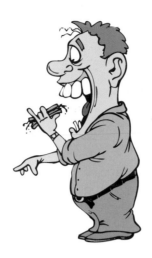

This is an expanding universe and we are all getting fatter. Last week's reports from health watchdogs had me reaching in a panic for the biscuit tin – just as I was about to eat every single Jaffa Cake, I knew I had to throw them all away. Comfort eating is over – actually eating is over. We had all better stop now, before it's too late.

In the US, 61% of adults are overweight. The average width of cinema and stadium seats has been increased from 17 inches to 22 inches – it will sound much worse when they go metric – and a woman weighing 60 stone (yes, 60) sued an airline who refused to let her on the plane because she couldn't be strapped into her seat.

American-style fat will soon become British fat, as we eat our way towards global parity on the scales. It's been called the 'McDonaldisation of diet', and the sad thing is that although Europe is our true neighbour, we prefer American eating habits. Burger and chips, Coke and crisps, convenience foods and heavily sauced ready meals have gobbled up the market for lean meat and veg and good, simple cooking. Why?

To call it a class issue is not enough. When I was growing up we were too poor to buy anything but raw ingredients and cook them. Meat twice a week may have led to some protein deficiencies, but meat twice a day, which is the average fast-food lifestyle, overloads the body with toxins as well as fat. The 'mechanically recovered' meat in pies and pasties is meat scraped off the animal carcass – it's not a cut, it's a kind of edible pulp fiction.

The fiction is that we are better off than our parents' generation, that everyone in the west is well nourished, and if we are a bit porky then, OK, it's better than starving.

The truth is that increasing numbers of people in the west are starving – that is, their bodies are chronically deprived of nutrients, but they are also fat. This is a brand-new problem in the world's horror list. We have reinvented malnutrition, and we are exporting our new disease.

Developing countries have traditionally struggled with famine and lack. Now they are struggling with famine and fat. In South Africa and Papua New Guinea, childhood malnutrition and adult obesity coexist; 70% of Samoans are now overweight. Countries whose chief health problems were infectious diseases and risk of famine must now cope with the diseases of affluence: cancer, heart conditions and diabetes.

No health service has the resources for a long-term epidemic of fat. Four children in Britain have now been diagnosed with an obesity-linked diabetes previously only found in adults over 40. Who is going to pay for their treatment? Well, we all are, but what when four becomes 4m, or 40m? Will Gordon Brown have to introduce a fat tax?

A fat tax could be levied, not on individuals but on fattening foods. Why not make chips the price of caviar? Of course anyone can buy spuds and make their own chips, but most people don't do that, they buy them in a bag, or they go down the chippy.

There are only two ways to halt the fast-food culture – make it expensive, and make the alternatives cheap. We could support farmers, we could support organics, we could reintroduce what used to be called domestic science into schools, and make it compulsory for boys and girls twice a week. We could bring back real school dinners and make them free. We could hire Nigella to impersonate the wartime cook Marguerite Patten and teach us all how to eat healthily using only a bag of mung beans, two fresh eggs and a sing-song round the piano.

What we can't do is to go on as we are. We can't afford to be fat. Fat food degrades the environment and it degrades us. Profit-driven factory food is turning human beings into gross parodies of themselves. We can't live in a world weighed down with greed and waste. We can't condemn our children to a life sentence in a prison of fat.

Before I get hundreds of heavy letters from the Right to Be Fat lobby, let me say that this is not about aesthetics, nor am I a secret member of the Fat Police. Fat is passive tissue and we are becoming a passive society, spoon-fed by faceless multinational interests, pacified on a diet of ready meals and TV.

Our bodies are a warning system – we should trust them. Don't we need to be a little bit hungry? Hungry for change, hungry for a fairer world? One thing is certain – a fairer world won't be a fatter world.

> *What we can't do is to go on as we are. We can't afford to be fat. Fat food degrades the environment and it degrades us*

Physical activity and obesity

Information from the Obesity Resource and Information Centre (ORIC)

People can become obese as a result of eating too much, not being sufficiently active, or both.

Traditionally, much more attention has been directed at dietary factors than low activity levels in the search for the cause of obesity and its treatment. Surprisingly, however, the recent rapid rise in obesity (from 6 to 15.5% in males and 8 to 16% in females) has occurred at a time when total energy intake and fat consumption have declined. At the same time, there have been steady but significant changes in our activity habits. There are fewer occupations requiring significant physical work. The affordability of the motor car and energy-saving devices at home and work, and the attractiveness and availability of home entertainment and computers have contributed to less active lifestyles. It has been estimated that our energy expenditure may have reduced by as much as 30%. It is clear from dietary surveys that reductions in energy intake have not kept pace with the fall in physical activity. The result is a rapid increase in the prevalence of obesity, especially in the lower socio-economic groups.

While it is often portrayed that we are becoming a fitness conscious society, national surveys indicate that this is only true for a small sector of the professional classes. Less than 20% of middle-aged and older adults are sufficiently active for health. Levels of activity in children have fallen as parents have become increasingly fearful of allowing them to play outdoors or walk or cycle to school. Only 5% of youngsters use their cycles as a form of transport in Britain as compared to 60-70% in Holland, and 30-40% of children are now taken to school by car, compared to 9% in 1971. English schools are at the bottom of the

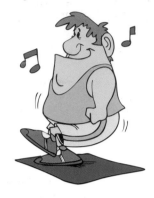

European league in terms of time allocated to physical education in primary and secondary schools, and school sport has declined in the last decade.

Definition of terms

Physical activity refers to all energy expended by movement or locomotion. This includes acts as mundane as walking, climbing stairs and gardening. Exercise is physical activity that is intentional and purposefully designed to improve some aspect(s) of fitness or health. It can include a walking programme, but can also mean more specific activities such as aerobic dance, weight training, and a range of sports. Even active pastimes such as gardening or line dancing can be considered exercise if the intention is to enhance health and well-being. Sport is a form of physical activity which involves structured competitive situations governed by rules. Physical fitness is a widely used term referring to a set of attributes such as strength and stamina that determine the individual's ability to undertake various types of activity.

Does physical activity help people lose weight?

Several recent reviews have considered the effect of exercise on weight loss. Although results from studies vary, the addition of exercise to a moderate diet provides a small increment in weight loss. A small weight loss is also found when exercise is not accompanied by a diet. Taken together, this research suggests that an exercise programme involving daily walking or three or four sessions of exercise per week

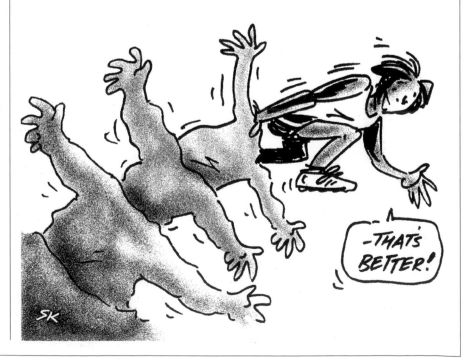

SK

—THAT'S BETTER!

will produce a weight loss of approximately 1kg (2lbs) per month in overweight to mildly obese people. Although this is small with respect to most dietary strategies, increased levels of exercise also have other benefits independent of weight loss.

Many studies have demonstrated that when exercise is combined with dietary restriction the proportion of weight lost as fat is greater than dieting alone. This is because exercise conserves or even develops muscle tissue, particularly if resistance (weight) training is used. Maintenance of muscle mass by exercise helps to preserve metabolic rate. In addition, exercise helps the individual who is losing weight feel firmer and more toned than if the weight loss is through diet alone, when the body is more likely to feel saggy and baggy. This can have a positive effect on motivation and body image and perhaps improve long-term outcomes. There are clear benefits of regular exercise for people trying to lose weight. However, exercise alone is more likely to play a critical role in long-term weight control for overweight and mildly obese individuals rather than the severely obese who often find it difficult to achieve significant levels of weight-bearing movement. However, as weight is lost by other methods, exercise levels can be gradually increased.

Men and women who walk regularly, or run, cycle, golf, or dance are less likely to gain weight than inactive individuals

---

Does physical activity help people keep weight off?

Helping people sustain their weight loss remains the major challenge in obesity treatment. Although there are many treatments for obesity, the long-term success is disappointing. Regular exercise appears to be an important component of weight-loss maintenance programmes. A recent

Summary

- Exercise assists weight loss and helps individuals retain muscle tissue and tone.
- Maintainance of regular exercise is very important for sustained weight loss.
- Physical activity greatly improves the chances of avoiding middle-age weight gain.
- Physical activity is very important to the health of the overweight and obese individual.

review showed that the average sustained weight loss over a minimum of 6 months was 4.0kg in 4 diet-only programmes, 4.9kg in 5 exercise-only programmes, and 7.2kg in 3 diet and exercise programmes. It is not fully established why exercise improves long-term weight loss. The extra energy expended only partially explains the effect. The maintenance of lean tissue may contribute. It is also possible that exercisers find additional motivation, either through improved body image, self-esteem, or a sense of personal control to better manage their lifestyles.

Can physical activity help prevent overweight and obesity?

Given the poor long-term success in the treatment of obesity, prevention is critical. In general, active people are slimmer than sedentary people. Men and women who walk regularly, or run, cycle, golf, or dance are less likely to gain weight than inactive individuals. One study shows that the chances of 13kg of weight gain over a 10-year period are 7 times higher in sedentary women than the active group, whilst sedentary men are 3.9 times more likely to gain 8-13kgs than men who report a high level of activity. Men or women who become inactive increase their risk of weight gain

© The Obesity Resource and Information Centre (ORIC)

Think-tank calls for unhealthy food tax

By Andrew Sparrow, Political Correspondent

Unhealthy food should be taxed, a left-wing think-tank will argue this week. Demos, which has close links with the Government, will urge ministers to consider imposing a levy on 'fatty, highly processed and fast foods' in order to encourage people to eat more healthily.

In a report that covers 'food poverty', Demos will point out that poor diet is to blame for health problems such as obesity and that this is a particular problem for low-income families, who are proportionally more likely to eat food with a high fat and sugar content.

The issue is contentious because food is exempt from value added tax and politicians in the past have been reluctant to consider putting a tax on such an essential commodity.

A Demos spokesman said: 'We are saying there should be some disincentive mechanism to tackle the issue of low cost, high fat, low nutrition food, which is bought disproportionally by low income people. But it has got to be done in a way that penalises the manufacturers, not the consumers.'

The spokesman added: 'It is vitally important that it does not just further penalise people who are already being penalised because they are forced into buying low nutrition food.'

The report, *Inconvenience Food*, will argue that any money raised from the tax should be used to encourage healthier eating habits. But it will not explain in detail how any of this could work.

Demos will launch its report in the Commons on Wednesday.

© Telegraph Group Limited, London 2002

Myths about physical activity

Information from the World Health Organization (WHO)

Being physically active is too expensive. It takes equipment, special shoes and clothes . . . and sometimes you even have to pay to use sports facilities.

Physical activity can be done almost anywhere and requires no equipment! Carrying groceries, wood, books or children are good complementary physical activities, as is climbing the stairs. Walking, perhaps the most practised and most highly recommended physical activity, is absolutely free. Most urban areas have some parks, waterfronts or other pedestrian areas that are ideal for walking, running or playing. There is no need to go to a gym, pool or other special sports facility to be physically active.

I'm very busy. Physical activity takes too much time!

At least thirty minutes of moderate physical activity every day are recommended to improve and maintain your health. This does not mean, however, that you must stop what you are doing and perform some physical activity for half an hour.

Most activities can be incorporated into your regular daily activities – at work, school, home or play. Also, the activity can be accumulated over the course of the day: a ten minute brisk walk, three times a day; or twenty minutes first thing in the morning and ten-minutes later in the day.

Even if you are very busy – you can still work in thirty minutes of activity into your daily routine.

Children by nature have so much energy. They hardly sit still. There's no need to spend time or energy teaching them about physical activity. They are already so active.

Recent studies have shown that children around the world are becoming increasingly sedentary – especially in poor urban areas. Time and resources devoted to physical education are being cut and computer games and television are replacing physically active pastimes. It is estimated that in many countries, both developed and developing, more than two-thirds of young people are insufficiently active. Inadequate physical activity in children can have lifelong health consequences.

Regular physical activity provides young people with important physical, mental and social health benefits. Being active has the potential to help children and young people develop coordination; build and maintain healthy bones, muscles and joints; control body weight and reduce fat; and develop efficient function of the heart and lungs. Play, games and other physical activities give young people opportunities for self-expression, building self-confidence, feelings of achievement, social interaction and integration. It also helps prevent and control feelings of anxiety and depression.

Involvement in properly guided physical activity and sports can also foster the adoption of other healthy behaviour including avoidance of tobacco, alcohol and drug use and violent behaviour. Patterns of physical activity acquired during childhood and adolescence are more likely to be maintained throughout the life span, thus providing the basis for active and healthy life. On the other hand, unhealthy lifestyles – including sedentary lifestyle, poor diet and substance abuse, adopted at a young age are likely to persist in adulthood.

Physical activity is for people in the 'prime of life'. At my age, I don't need to be concerned with it . . .

Physical activity can improve quality of life in many ways for people of all ages. Active lifestyles provide older persons with regular occasions to

> *Physical activity can improve quality of life in many ways for people of all ages*

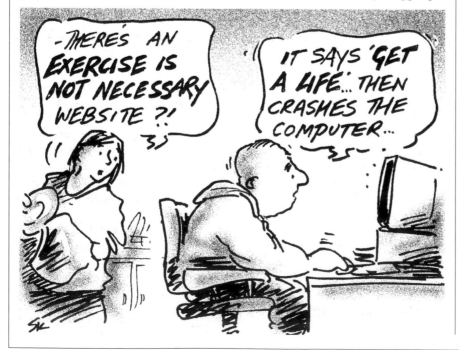

make new friendships, maintain social networks, and interact with other people of all ages. Improved flexibility, balance, and muscle tone can help prevent falls – a major cause of disability among older people. It has been found that the prevalence of mental illness is lower among people who are physically active.

Physical activity can also contribute greatly to the management of some mental disorders such as depression. Organised exercise sessions, appropriately suited to an individual's fitness level, or simply casual walks can provide the opportunity for making new friends and maintaining ties with the community, reducing feelings of loneliness and social exclusion. Physical activity can also help to improve self-confidence and self-sufficiency – qualities that are the foundation of psychological well-being.

The benefits of physical activity can be enjoyed even if regular practice starts late in life

The benefits of physical activity can be enjoyed even if regular practice starts late in life. While being active from an early age can help prevent many diseases, regular movement and activity can also help relieve the disability and pain associated with common diseases among older people including arthritis, osteoporosis, and hypertension.

Physical activity is needed only in industrialised countries. Developing countries have other problems.

The lack of physical activity is a major underlying cause of death, disease, and disability. Preliminary data from a WHO study on risk factors suggest that inactivity, or sedentary lifestyle, is one of the 10 leading global causes of death and disability. More than two million deaths each year are attributable to physical inactivity. In countries around the world between 60% and 85% of adults are simply not active enough to benefit their health.

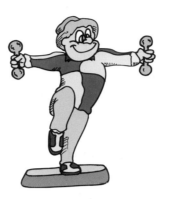

Sedentary lifestyles increase all causes of mortality, double the risk of cardiovascular diseases, diabetes, and obesity, and substantially increase the risks of colon cancer, high blood pressure, osteoporosis, depression and anxiety.

In the rapidly growing cities of the developing world, crowding, poverty, crime, traffic, poor air quality, a lack of parks, sidewalks, sports and recreation facilities and other safe areas make physical activity a difficult choice. For example, in São Paulo, Brazil, 70% of the population is inactive. Even in rural areas of developing countries sedentary pastimes such as watching television are increasingly popular. In addition to other lifestyle changes, the consequences are growing levels of obesity, diabetes, and cardiovascular diseases.

Low- and middle-income countries suffer the greatest impact from these and other noncommunicable diseases – 77% of the total number of deaths caused by noncommunicable diseases occur in developing countries. These diseases are on the rise. They will have an increasingly severe effect on health care systems, resources, and economies in countries around the world.

These countries are struggling to manage the impact of infectious diseases simultaneously with the growing burden on society and health systems caused by noncommunicable diseases. Physical activity, in addition to healthy diet and smoke-free lifestyle, is an efficient, cost-effective and sustainable way for promoting public health in low- and middle-income countries.

■ The above information is from the World Health Organization's web site which can be found at www.who.int

© 2002 WHO/OMS

Fears for 'generation of couch potatoes'

More than a fifth of Scots are obese and the trend is rising rapidly among children, according to a report released yesterday by Scotland's chief medical officer.

Dr Mac Armstrong found that nearly eight per cent of boys and seven per cent of girls were classed as obese. Dr Armstrong said: 'The increasing levels of obesity in Scottish children and the subsequent health implications for later life are of concern.'

He said type 2 diabetes, traditionally seen in the over-40s and associated with obesity, poor diet and lack of exercise, was being found in children as young as 13.

He also highlighted the lack of exercise among Scots, with six out of 10 men and seven out of 10 women estimated to be taking less than the recommended levels of physical activity.

'This is the generation of couch potatoes and the bad news for our future is that these bad habits are being learnt by younger people,' said Dr Armstrong.

Although he estimated that 500,000 Scots had coronary heart disease, with a further 180,000 showing symptoms, he revealed that cancer had overtaken it as the main cause of death.

Lung cancer was the most common cause of death among cancers, and Dr Armstrong said 34 per cent of Scots men smoked and 32 per cent of women, among the highest rates in Europe.

© Telegraph Group Limited, London 2002

The obesity pandemic

Will parents outlive their children?

By Andrew Prentice,
Professor of International
Nutrition

In affluent nations obesity has been the fastest growing health epidemic for the past two decades. Many nations now record over 20% of their adult population as clinically obese and well over half the population as overweight. The epidemic struck first in the USA and is spreading rapidly outwards. High levels of obesity are now recorded in Europe (especially Eastern Europe), Australasia, Central America and the Middle East. Asian nations are reporting rapid increases in their statistics (albeit from a low baseline) and some of the poorest nations in the world have burgeoning levels of obesity in their urban areas. Thus the original epidemic in North America can now be described as a pandemic.

These remarkable changes in the shape and anatomical composition of mankind represent a 'grade shift' in our evolution caused by a sudden change in the external environment in which we now live (abundant high-energy foods and a reduction in energy output caused by the technological revolution of the late 20th century). The last such shift in our shape occurred about 2 centuries ago in Europe and involved an increase in average adult height by 30cm or more. This change in height is generally viewed as being beneficial since tallness is generally associated with better health outcomes (except for some cancers which are more common in taller people). However, the recent increase in girth is associated with a host of very damaging health outcomes which may undermine much of the progress that has been made in the last century in terms of health and longevity.

Obesity is a powerful risk factor for a host of diseases ranging from relatively minor ailments (breathlessness and exercise intolerance, varicose veins and many others) through quite serious conditions (osteoarthritis, back pain, hypertension, etc.) to conditions that are frequently fatal (diabetes, stroke, coronary heart disease, sleep apnoea and cancer). The association with type 2 diabetes is particularly powerful with obese women up to 100 times more likely to suffer than lean women and obese men up to 45 times more likely.

> *As things stand the prognostications are not good. If anything, the obesity pandemic is gathering pace rather than slowing down, and current interventions are only marginally effective and very expensive*

Diabetes then acts as a precipitator of a spectrum of other serious conditions which in turn shorten lifespan.

So, will parents outlive their children as claimed recently by an American obesity specialist? The answer is yes – and no. Yes, when the offspring become grossly obese. This is now becoming an alarmingly common occurrence in the US, and type 2 diabetes (once described as 'adult onset obesity') is now being reported from paediatric clinics. Such children and adolescents have a greatly reduced quality of life in terms of both their physical and psychosocial health. The accumulation of chronic diseases precipitated by their obesity predicts a considerable shortening of lifespan (recently estimated to average 9 years for clinically obese people and likely to be much more in the severely obese).

On a population-wide basis the answer to whether parents (as a generation) will outlive their children depends on the extent to which we continue to get fatter and on the success of, and willingness to invest in, medical and pharmacological interventions to combat the ill effects of obesity. As things stand the prognostications are not good. If anything the obesity pandemic is gathering pace rather than slowing down, and current interventions are only marginally effective and very expensive. Reliance on medical interventions to combat obesity would require highly costly lifelong treatments administered to over half the population.

■ The above article is from a press release by the London School of Hygiene and Tropical Medicine.

© Andrew Prentice, London School of Hygiene and Tropical Medicine

Couch potato lifestyle

Couch potato lifestyle is worse for your health than smoking. By Celia Hall

Poor diet and lack of exercise cause more illness than smoking, new figures show.

The lifestyle of couch potatoes has overtaken smoking as the major cause of ill-health in EU countries for the first time, the World Health Organization says.

Dr Aileen Robertson told the European Society of Cardiology annual meeting in Berlin yesterday that doctors and governments must take the issue of diet and exercise more seriously.

Telling people to eat more fruit and vegetables and to take exercise did not work if there were no policies to help people change, she said.

'I am not saying that smoking plays no part in ill-health. I am saying that diet is as important and we have to get that through because it is not understood at the moment.'

Dr Robertson, a regional adviser for nutrition at the WHO in Copenhagen, said that Japan had the highest rates of smoking in the world but also the lowest rates of heart disease.

She criticised the EU for discouraging farmers from growing the healthiest food. Europe did not produce enough fruit and vegetables for everyone to eat five portions a day, as the WHO recommended.

'In Spain, Greece and Italy they grow a surplus of fruit and vegetables, but millions of tons are destroyed every year to maintain the market price.

'It is possible to produce enough fruit and vegetables for all of Europe to follow the recommendations by spreading the fresh food across the countries, but current policies do not support this.'

The WHO study shows that smoking causes nine per cent of all chronic diseases in the EU, while physical inactivity and diet are responsible for 9.7 per cent.

The main conditions caused by bad diet are heart disease, followed by cancer.

> **The lifestyle of couch potatoes has overtaken smoking as the major cause of ill-health in EU countries for the first time**

'Around 30 to 40 per cent of cancer cases could be prevented through better diet,' Dr Robertson said.

'Obesity in adults is up 20 to 30 per cent and is also escalating among children, increasing their future risk of cardiovascular disease.'

Dr Robertson gave examples of programmes in Finland which had reduced heart disease by 65 per cent between 1972 and 1994.

They included paying farmers to switch from dairy to berry farming.

Councils were encouraged to include fruit and vegetables in employees' packed lunches.

There were also new food labelling projects and diet guidelines for all food provided in schools, hospitals and places of work.

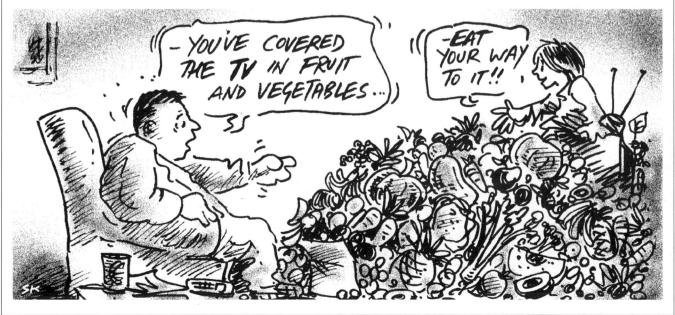

Jonah Lomu is fat . . .

. . . according to the official method of measuring obesity, the body mass index. There must be a better way, says Michael Hann

You may have read with a shudder last week's horror stories about obesity: the news that our kids are getting so fat that they might die before us, and that a 'silent epidemic' of weight gain is set to overtake smoking as the biggest cause of preventable death. All over the land, people will have been furtively hitting the calculator keys to work out their body mass index (BMI) and see if they, too, were classified as obese.

Well, that shudder may have been a little premature, because in individual cases the formula is not as helpful as you might believe. The BMI, a method used worldwide to determine how healthy a person's weight is, is based on the relationship between an individual's height and weight. At a reading of 25 or above, you are overweight. But so, according to the calculations, is Mel Gibson. And at 30, you become obese; but so are Arnold Schwarzenegger, Jonah Lomu and Sylvester Stallone.

The simplicity of the BMI makes it a godsend for looking at trends. But it is also something of a broad-brush tool. It takes no account of age, sex or race; it makes no allowance for your fitness. Most importantly, it does not measure how much fat you are carrying or how that fat is distributed.

Professor Ian Macdonald, co-editor of the *International Journal of Obesity*, explains that the fat you need to worry about is abdominal fat. Fat above the hips puts a strain on your heart, putting you at risk. Below the hips, it is not such a problem.

The system also fails to take into account the amount of fat you are carrying – hence the reason for the 'obesity' of Jonah, Arnie and Sly. Dense, muscled physiques can weigh more than flabby, unfit ones, with the result that the superfit can end up being categorised as obese.

So why don't doctors measure a patient's body fat before pronouncing on their weight? Because they have neither the time nor the resources, says Macdonald.

> *At a reading of 25 or above, you are overweight. But so, according to the calculations, is Mel Gibson. And at 30, you become obese; but so are Jonah Lomu and Sylvester Stallone*

Furthermore, the measurements given by the fitness-club favourite – the skin callipers – should also be treated with care. 'Skin callipers are very useful when done properly,' says Macdonald. 'But it depends on the experience and skill of the person using them.' He says a week of training is necessary before someone can use callipers properly – which is four and three-quarters more days than the fitness assessor is likely to have had before they pronounce you flabby.

But even getting an accurate assessment of your body-fat level might not be helpful in determining how much weight you need to lose. A study in the *American Journal of Clinical Nutrition* in 2000 found that healthy body-fat levels vary by age, gender and race. So a white man in his early 20s might have a healthy range of 8% to 21% body fat, while for a black woman aged between 60 and 79 the healthy range is between 23% and 35%. The BMI takes no notice of such distinctions: GPs in this country work to a measure designed for western Europeans, yet inner-city general practice lists are becoming increasingly multi-ethnic. Other parts of the world are thinking of altering their BMI charts to take account of their different physiques.

The BMI is also problematic

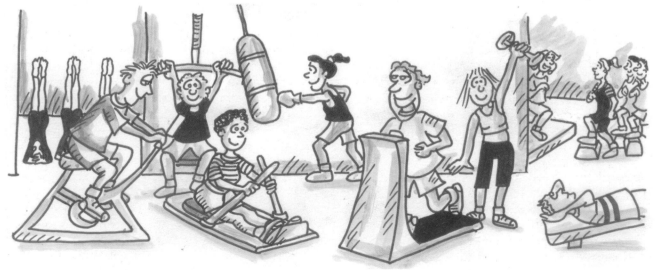

when used on children. Although specialist clinics will almost certainly have child-specific BMI tables, the chances are your GP won't. And the easy-reference charts that you can find on the internet are certainly not designed for children.

Being classified as obese under the BMI can damage more than your self-esteem. Julia, a 27-year-old who ate healthily and exercised regularly, was told by the nurse at her GP's surgery that she was obese at 5ft 9in and 83kg. 'She told me I was fat and 71kg was the most I should weigh.'

There is an easy and simple alternative: look at your waist size. For men, a waist size of more than 91cm (36in) should give you cause for concern, the equivalent figure for women is 80cm (32.5in)

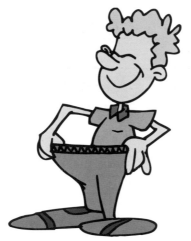

Julia started to live on a diet of crispbread, stir-fries and baked beans. She went to the gym or ran every day. She started to throw up any significant meal she ate. 'I got down to 71kg in about 10 weeks but it stopped there,' she says. 'I just couldn't lose any more, and my friends told me I was looking gaunt.' Julia, who has now put weight back on, realised she had developed an eating disorder because her weight was expressed to her only as a function of her BMI.

Such simplistic advice is all too common, says Dr Ian Campbell, chairman of the National Obesity Forum. He says that too many health professionals in this country do not understand that a healthy weight is about more than a BMI reading. 'I've been on a personal crusade about it,' he says. 'But it's what doctors in this country have always been taught.'

Campbell, Macdonald and others say there is an easy and simple alternative: look at your waist size. For men, a waist size of more than 91cm (36in) should give you cause for concern. More than 101cm (40in) and you need to lose weight urgently. The equivalent figures for women are 80cm (32.5in) and 88cm (34.5in). By this criterion, Lomu, with his 27in waist, kicks the obesity tag into touch.

Macdonald, though, offers a word of caution to those who think this gives them an excuse to avoid that trip to the gym: 'You can't get away with saying, "I've got a big frame, so this doesn't apply to me." It does.'

© *Guardian Newspapers Limited 2002*

Wise up to your waist size

Says the British Dietetic Association

Around 1 in 5 men and 1 in 3 women are currently trying to lose weight, according to a recent nationwide ICM Research poll commissioned by the British Dietetic Association (BDA). Throughout June, the BDA will be asking the nation to wise up to its waist size as it launches a new national campaign, Weight Wise. The campaign, which forms part of its annual Food First programme, aims to raise awareness of the benefits of a balanced and varied diet in achieving and maintaining a healthy weight.

'Obesity is one of the most serious public health problems in the UK today. About 1 in 5 adults are heavy enough to be putting their health at risk – increasing the chance of having a heart attack, developing diabetes or having a high blood pressure,' said Dr Helen Lloyd, a spokesperson from the British Dietetic Association. 'Having excess body fat around the waist compared with around the hips can be particularly unhealthy,' she added.

A waist circumference measurement of more than 32 inches (80cm) for a woman and 37 inches (94cm) for a man increases health risks.

The research poll revealed that only around 6 out of 10 adults were aware that it is more dangerous to your health to carry extra weight around your waist. However, the same survey revealed that most people are fairly knowledgeable when it comes to approaches to losing weight. When asked what they would consider to be a healthy and successful approach to losing weight, 9 out of 10 adults agreed with choosing healthy eating and being more active and two-thirds would consult a health professional. Fortunately, just around 1 in 4 considered food combining diets to be a good method, with similar numbers reporting a detox programme to be a healthy and successful approach. When asked which nutrient to cut down on most in the diet to lose or control body weight, just over 6 out of 10 respondents correctly identified fat.

Throughout June (Food First month) State Registered Dietitians will be working with members of the public across the UK to raise awareness of the benefits of being a healthy weight and offering ideas and practical help on safe and effective weight management.

■ The above information is from the British Dietetic Association's web site which can be found at www.bda.uk.com

© *British Dietetic Association*

Britons stand tall, if slightly heavy, in Europe

By John Carvel, Social Affairs Editor

Not every European dimension has been harmonised in Brussels yet. According to the Department for Trade and Industry, the average Briton stands head, shoulders, girth and bottoms above their continental partners.

The figures come in a new edition of the department's handbook of anthropometric and strength measurements, compiled by ergonomists at the University of Nottingham to help manufacturers design products to fit people's shape.

The volume provides 294 measurements ranging from the distance between the inner corners of the eyes to the length of the leg between the crease below the buttock and the crease at the back of the knee.

It has discovered that the average British man is 36 millimetres (1 inch) taller than his French counterpart.

The mean height of UK citizens is 1,755.1mm (5ft 9in). Among European men only the Dutch are taller, averaging 1,795mm and with a clear height advantage over the US men's average of 1,760.4.

The average British woman is 1,620mm tall (just under 5ft 4in), compared with 1,604mm for her French counterpart, 1,610mm for the Italians and 1,619mm for the Germans. Swedish women average 1,640mm, Dutch 1,650mm and Americans 1,626.7mm.

More disturbingly, British men and women are heavier than all the other nationalities except the Americans, averaging 79.75 kilos for British men and 66.7 for women.

The average British woman has a chest measurement of 1,007.8mm (39.7 inches), compared with 965mm for the Italians, 912.6mm for the Japanese and 806mm for Sri Lankans. American women also top this scale with an average of 1,047.2mm.

The average British woman's waist is 840.6mm (33 inches) – also second largest behind the Americans. But her bottom at 873.7mm is considerably smaller than the Italians at 916mm who beat the Americans into second place.

The average British male foot is 266.8mm long (10.5 inches), 6mm longer than the French and Germans, 3mm more than the Italians and 1mm more than the Swedes. But they are just beaten by the Americans at 267.8mm and massively outstripped by the Dutch at 275mm.

> *British men and women are heavier than all the other nationalities except the Americans, averaging 79.75 kilos for British men and 66.7 for women*

However Dutch women have daintier feet than the British, averaging 240mm compared with 241.1mm in the UK (9.5 inches). German women average 242mm, compared with 245mm for the Swedes and 242.1mm for the Americans.

The DTI has a less than exhaustive record of ring finger lengths, but on the available evidence the British man's finger at 78.7mm (3.1 inches) is 1.7mm longer than his German counterpart, but 0.2mm shorter than the American average.

The British woman's ring finger at 72.6mm is 0.4mm smaller than her German counterpart and 0.3mm smaller than the American.

Beverley Norris, research fellow at Nottingham university's institute for occupational ergonomics, said the figures were useful for product designers.

The department has recently completed a study of the pulling force needed to open ring-pull cans.

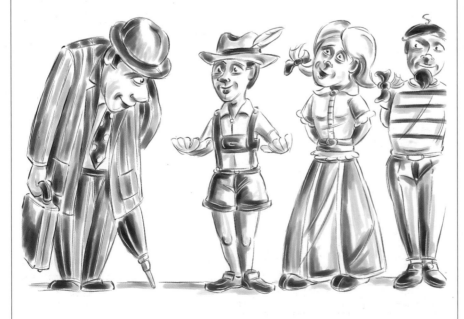

Diet industry

Diet industry will be winner in battle of the bulge as Europe goes to fat

A tide of obesity will sweep Europe over the next four years and cause a boom in the diet industry as consumers try to get back into shape, market analysts said yesterday. The most serious weight problems will be seen in Germany where the proportion of people who are overweight or obese will increase from 57% last year to 71% in 2006.

Problems of excess weight will affect 69% of adults in Spain and the Netherlands, 60% of Swedes and 59% of Italians.

Although Britain and France will have weight problems, they will have more people who are underweight than obese.

In Britain the proportion who are overweight or obese will increase from 48% last year to 52% in 2006. In France it will rise from 37% to 50%.

The forecasts were prepared by the market analysts Datamonitor on the basis of trends since 1996. Obesity was measured using a body mass index to measure excess fat. The index divides the person's weight in kilograms by their height in metres squared. A BMI of 20-25 is normal, 25-30 is overweight and more than 30 is obese.

By John Carvel, Social Affairs Editor

Andrew Russell, the company's consumer market analyst, said the trend to excess weight followed 20 years of convenience foods and unconventional mealtimes.

'Modern diets are more calorific, yet people expend less energy during the day . . . Those who find themselves overweight and those who are keen to avoid being in that position are increasingly interested in using both exercise and diet to manage their shape,' he said.

The diet food and drinks market would increase from £51bn in 1996 to £61bn in 2006.

The underweight were the least likely to take exercise, but people of normal weight were 'a good market segment as they display a strong desire to manage their shape and more willpower to apply the necessary changes to their lifestyle,' he said.

The overweight were the second most profitable group. They would continually try to make small changes to their lifestyle and diet without ever removing the underlying need

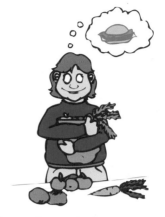

to do so. This made them 'potentially lifelong customers'.

'While both the normal weight and overweight consumer can oscillate between a desire for health and a desire for indulgence, the overweight consumer will do so with greater frequency – possibly even between lunchtime and dinner.'

Mr Russell said people abstaining from alcohol because they were concerned about their weight or shape would cost the European drinks industry £3.2bn by 2006.

In Britain the proportion who are overweight or obese will increase from 48% last year to 52% in 2006. In France it will rise from 37% to 50%.

■ Children are 'eating themselves sick' with poor diets and unhealthy lifestyles, nutritionists warned yesterday during a conference at the Royal College of Paediatrics and Child Health in London. They suggested that postwar rationing was better for children than the 21st-century snack culture.

Youngsters today were experiencing the nutritional equivalent of the Victorian age when rickets and scurvy were commonplace.

© *Guardian Newspapers Limited 2002*

Activity in schools

The European Survey in 1993 showed that secondary schools in England and Wales allocate less time to PE than anywhere else in Europe. Since then, the situation in England has become worse with the proportion of children spending two, or more hours per week in school sport decreasing from 46% in 1994 to 33% in 1999.[1]

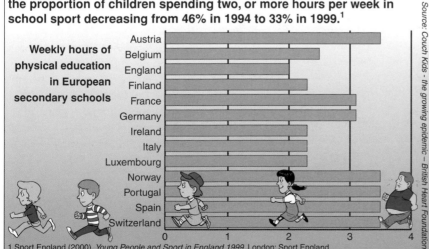

Weekly hours of physical education in European secondary schools

Source: Couch Kids - the growing epidemic – British Heart Foundation

1 Sport England (2000). *Young People and Sport in England 1999*. London: Sport England

Nutrition news

Reading between the headlines

Hardly a day goes by when a story about nutrition or diet doesn't hit the newsstands. Whether it's a new 'food scare' or the latest Hollywood diet, nutrition stories make good headlines. And with good reason, because what we eat and drink is something that affects every one of us. While it can sometimes be difficult to demystify the jargon and try to identify what, if any, changes we need to make to improve our health and well-being, there are ways to help identify whether the information is science-based and relevant to you.

While family, friends and books are all important, the main sources of information on nutrition today are the media and the Internet. The scores of magazines, newspapers, television and radio programmes and the huge variety of websites on diet and health provide a wealth of information. A lot of good information based on sound science is available. However, sometimes information on diet and food safety can be oversimplified, lack context or even be downright inaccurate. So how can you tell one from the other?

The table below provides some valuable tips for helping to identify if information about science, including nutrition and food safety, is questionable. Claims that sound 'too good to be true' and listing foods as 'good' or 'bad' are some of the warning signs that the information needs careful scrutiny.

Simplifying information

Writers and journalists need to simplify information so that it can

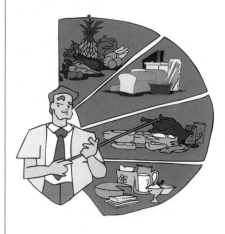

be delivered in the context of a story or article. This simplification can sometimes lead to important information being overlooked. For example, stories may fail to place the finding into context or do not include background information. These factors are important considerations when determining whether or not the information relates to you, especially if the story reports on new scientific findings. For example, if a study in Japanese men showed that eating seaweed five times a week prevented cancer, do the findings relate to you? Perhaps and perhaps not. You need to look at how studies are conducted and in which population groups including nationalities, ages and race. Look at the number of people in the study – generally, the larger the number, the more reliable the results. Also check if the results agree with those found by other studies.

It is also important to check the source of the information. Has the study been published in a reputable journal? Has it been reviewed by experts in the area to ensure that it followed scientific procedures and was properly executed? Is the writer credible? Does the report or study agree with recommendations from credible professional agencies or government departments?

The Internet is an area where careful scrutiny of information is especially warranted. Anyone can set up a site on the Internet and cyberspace is littered with misinformation, fraud and quackery. While good science-based informa-

tion does exist, some sites are just advertisements to sell particular products or to promote the agendas of political and ideological groups.

Recommendations don't change overnight

Remember that nutrition research, like most other areas of research, is evolutionary. Recommendations on healthy lifestyles don't change overnight. They need to be based on many scientific studies, rigorously conducted and repeated over time in many different groups and reviewed and debated by scientists. A healthy dose of scepticism coupled with common sense and checking with credible authorities is the best way to approach food and nutrition news.

The Ten Red Flags of Junk Science

Be careful if the information contains:

- Recommendations that promise a quick fix.
- Dire warnings of danger from a single product or regime.
- Claims that sound too good to be true.
- Simplistic conclusions drawn from a complex study.
- Recommendations based on a single study.
- Dramatic statements that are refuted by reputable scientific organisations.
- Lists of 'good' and 'bad' foods.
- Recommendations made to help sell a product.
- Recommendations based on studies published without peer review.
- Recommendations from studies that ignore differences among individuals or groups.

■ The above information is from the European Food Information Council's (EUFIC) web site which can be found at www.eufic.org

© 2002, EUFIC

The benefits of exercise

Information from Absolute Fitness

Physical benefits

It's a question that has gone through everyone's mind from time to time – Why bother? Wouldn't I be happier lifting a pint instead of this dumb-bell? Why am I running in the rain instead of (insert your favourite pastime here) – am I mad?!

But there's a good reason why you are putting yourself through your paces. In fact, there are hundreds of good reasons, and we all know what they are – we just need reminding from time to time.

One of the biggest killers of the modern age is lack of exercise. It's as simple as that. By taking even moderate exercise on a regular basis our immune system is strengthened – and we cut the risk of heart disease, stroke, blood vessel disorders, thrombosis, angina; the list goes on. The key word here is regular: all exercise is good, but regular moderate exercise has a greater effect on your overall health than occasional bursts of lung-busting activity. In short, be as active as you can, as often as possible – and KEEP IT GOING!!!

Life just seems much easier when you are fit – and it's not just the body that benefits from exercise. Exercise triggers chemical changes in the brain that can have a powerful and positive effect on mental health.

The ability to deal with the daily demands of hard work and play more effectively is one of the most underestimated side effects of fitness – and one of the best!

Psychological benefits

The psychological benefits of regular exercise can be as significant as the physical. Some, such as better self-esteem, come as an indirect result of exercise and are fairly subjective.

Others are a direct consequence of chemical activity triggered by physical exertion – for example,

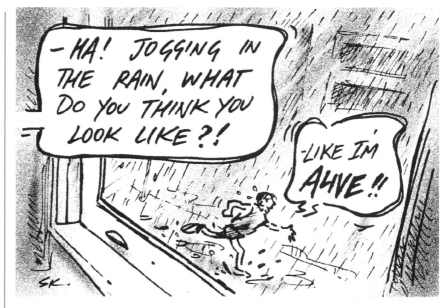

people suffering from depression or anxiety are often 'prescribed' exercise. Brain chemicals released during exercise, such as serotonin, dopamine, norepinephrine, and endorphins, are known to have strong effects on mood, helping reduce feelings of anxiety, stress and depression, while also helping to strengthen your immune system.

Twenty different types of endorphin have been discovered in the nervous system, and the beta-endorphins secreted during exercise have the most powerful effect. Sometimes described as 'runners high', the release of beta-endorphins reduces pain (the reason why running becomes easier after about 20 minutes) and stimulates feelings of euphoria – which is why so many people feel invigorated and enthusiastic after exercise.

Other psychological side effects of exercise include:
- Improved self-esteem and greater sense of self-reliance and self-confidence
- Improved mental alertness, perception and information processing

- Increased perceptions of acceptance by others
- Decreased overall feelings of stress and tension
- Reduced frustration with daily problems, and a more constructive response to disappointments and failures

These psychological benefits can be just as important as the more obvious physical ones; most of us exercise in the first place because we are unhappy about something, whether it is that spare tyre, worries about general health, or just being sick of feeling tired and unfit.

If you are feeling like a couch potato, or you are finding stress and worry is becoming a problem, get out there and exercise! The hardest part by far is that initial step, when it can feel like exercise is the last thing in the world that will cheer you up: try to remember that exercise is one of the very best ways to do just that.

■ The above information is from the Absolute Fitness web site: www.absolutefitness.co.uk

© Absolute Fitness

Be weight wise – be active

Information from the British Dietetic Association

Regular physical activity has a wealth of benefits, but today most of us tend to be quite inactive. We live in a 'push-button culture' full of labour-saving devices. Computers, video games, cars, escalators and automatic doors all result in our being increasingly inactive. Regular physical activity can improve your overall health and help prevent disease. Combined with healthy eating habits, regular physical activity is a great way to help you to lose or control your weight.

Why get active?

Being active helps you:
- Lose weight
- Maintain your weight loss
- Live longer, more healthily
- Keep your bones, muscles and joints healthy
- Improve your mood and reduce symptoms of anxiety and depression

Exercise also reduces your risk of:
- Dying from coronary heart disease
- Developing diabetes, colon cancer and high blood pressure

What activity should I do?

Anything you enjoy at a time you enjoy doing it. After all, if you don't enjoy it you probably won't do it. Or you'll start and then give up. You may enjoy team or group sports such as football or aerobics, or you may prefer individual activities such as swimming or walking. If you are a morning person then choose to do things in the morning when you have more energy.

There are basically two types of exercise: cardiovascular (aerobic) and resistance (weight) training.

Cardiovascular training includes anything that works your heart and lungs hard, such as brisk walking, jogging, swimming and cycling.

Resistance training includes the use of weights and machines. In an aquarobics class, the water acts as resistance and so this form of exercise could be a good one to choose as an alternative to training in a gym.

How often and how much activity should I do?

Be as active as possible as often as you can. Any amount of physical activity is better than none at all, and if you're already active your health will benefit from doing more. As a guide, try to do 30 minutes (or more) of moderate-intensity physical activity e.g. walking, swimming, housework or gardening every day.

Do you make any of the following excuses?

- 'I don't have time' – exercise doesn't have to be time-consuming. Just ten minutes every day can lead to health benefits.
- 'I'm too old' – anyone can get active at any age.
- 'It's expensive' – not necessarily. You don't have to join a gym and you don't have to invest in expensive equipment.
- 'It's boring' – then find something that you enjoy. Dancing round when you're vacuuming can be just as beneficial as working out.
- 'It's dangerous' – it's certainly more dangerous if you don't exercise. But if you're worried, check with your GP first!

Top tips to get more active

- Clean the house with vigour
- Get up to change the TV channel
- Wash your car by hand
- Climb the stairs briskly
- Mow the lawn & rake the leaves
- Use the stairs, not the lift or escalator
- Go for a brisk walk

Vary your activities and remember to stretch and strengthen.

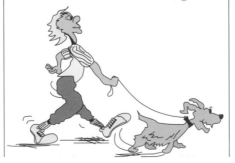

Variety is the spice of life – try different activities to stop yourself getting bored. Stretching and weight training should also be part of your regular exercise routine to help strengthen your bones and muscles, help to prevent injury, and use extra calories.

Find an exercise buddy

It's much more fun if you do things with friends and family. Go for a walk with a friend, play in the park with the kids, arrange to meet someone for a swim.

'But I never lose weight, however hard I try . . . '
Even so, eating healthily and taking regular exercise will still benefit you!

Safety tips

- Check with your doctor before you start exercising if you:
  - have ever been told you have heart problems or high blood pressure
  - have bone or joint problems that may be aggravated by exercise
  - are over the age of 65 and inactive
  - are on prescription medication
  - think that you may have any other reason for not exercising
- Dress appropriately – whether you are walking the dog or going to the gym, wear comfortable clothes.
- Invest in appropriate footwear e.g. trainers for walking and jogging.
- Start gradually and exercise at a comfortable pace.
- Always carry a drink with you.

- This information was produced by the British Dietetic Association as a factsheet for Food First 2002. The British Dietetic Association is the professional association for State Registered Dietitians. For more information on the British Dietetic Association and its Food First campaign visit www.bda.uk.com

© British Dietetic Association

Why exercise is wise

Information from www.KidsHealth.org

'Come on!' your gym teacher bellows. 'Just one more lap!' 'Why don't you head outside – it's a beautiful day, perfect for getting some exercise,' your mom says.

'Well, he seems to be in great shape. Give him these heartworm pills once a month and take him out for lots of exercise,' the vet says while looking over your new dog.

Exercise is a word you hear everywhere – and for good reason. Exercise is a very important part of life because it keeps the body in good shape (and not just in humans either, as the vet's comment shows). Doctors and researchers are finding evidence that regular exercise, along with other things that make up a healthy lifestyle, can prevent some diseases that occur later in life and lead to a longer, happier life in general.

Rewards and benefits

'So what? How does that affect me?' you may be thinking. Well, exercise doesn't just offer rewards when you're older – it offers rewards that begin right at this moment, too. Exercise is beneficial to every part of your body, including your brain. But probably the best place to start is your heart.

You most likely already know that the heart is a muscle – it's actually the strongest muscle in the human body. But did you know that just like other muscles, the heart likes (and needs) a good workout? You can provide it with an excellent workout in the form of aerobic exercise. Aerobic exercise is any type of exercise that makes your muscles use oxygen. Because aerobic exercise is repetitive, it brings fresh oxygen into the muscles of the body over and over – making the heart muscle stronger (and sometimes a bit larger, as well). Aerobic exercise increases the number of blood cells in your blood, so your blood can carry more oxygen than before; it also helps the blood travel more efficiently through your blood vessels.

It's recommended that teens do some sort of aerobic exercise at least three times a week, for 20 to 30 minutes at a time. Many teens who play team sports may do more than what's recommended – and that's great! The heart appreciates it and you'll be able to do more and more exercise without getting tired. Some team sports that are good for pouring on the oxygen are swimming, basketball, soccer, lacrosse, field hockey, ice and roller hockey, and rowing.

Regular exercise, along with other things that make up a healthy lifestyle, can prevent some diseases that occur later in life and lead to a longer, happier life in general

---

But if you don't play team sports, don't worry; there are plenty of ways to get aerobic exercise on your own or with a few friends. Some awesome ways to get aerobically fit include biking, running, aerobics, swimming, dancing, in-line skating, cross-country skiing, hiking, and walking quickly. In fact, types of exercise that you can do on your own are easier to continue for years to come, so you can stay fit as you get older.

The heart isn't the only muscle to benefit from regular exercise – most of the other muscles in your body enjoy exercise, too. Exercise makes muscles stronger and sometimes bigger. When muscles get built up and become stronger, it allows you to be active for longer periods of time without getting worn out. Strong muscles are also a plus because they actually help protect you when you exercise – they provide support to your joints and can help prevent injuries.

■ This information was provided by KidsHealth, one of the largest resources online for medically reviewed health information written for parents, kids, and teens. For more articles like this one, visit www.KidsHealth.org or www.TeensHealth.org

© KidsHealth

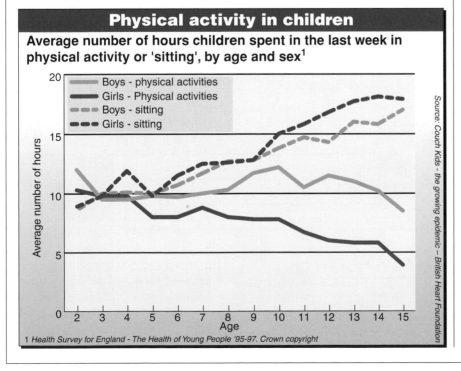

Physical activity in children

Average number of hours children spent in the last week in physical activity or 'sitting', by age and sex[1]

Legend:
- Boys - physical activities
- Girls - Physical activities
- Boys - sitting
- Girls - sitting

Y-axis: Average number of hours (0 to 20)
X-axis: Age (2 to 15)

Source: Couch Kids - the growing epidemic – British Heart Foundation

[1] Health Survey for England - The Health of Young People '95-97. Crown copyright

Exercise and your heart

Information from the Coronary Prevention Group

The human body was designed for an active life but these days we spend most of our time sitting down at our desks, watching TV, in our cars . . . Taking regular exercise helps keep you generally fit and healthy and regular exercise is essential for a healthy heart.

How exercise helps your heart . . .

It has been known for a long time that those who take regular physical activity either as part of their work (e.g. postmen) or in their leisure time, are less likely to have a heart attack then those who don't. Those who do not exercise regularly are more than twice as likely to have a heart attack than those who do.

Taking regular, adequate exercise helps to protect you from coronary heart disease because:

- Exercise builds up the strength of your heart so it can do its normal job of pumping blood around the body effortlessly. It also gives your heart more 'reserve capacity' so it is better able to cope when you ask it to pump harder!
- Exercise will help ensure that your blood pressure remains lower or help lower it if it is high.
- Exercise keeps the blood healthy by increasing levels of HDL, the 'good' cholesterol which helps clear cholesterol from the blood and it also makes the blood less likely to clot.
- Exercise helps to keep your weight in check.

. . . and your general health

As we get older, our bones lose calcium and become weaker. This is called osteoporosis and is more marked in women after the menopause. Taking regular exercise slows down that loss of calcium and keeps the bones stronger for longer.

Exercise is particularly good for older people as it keeps the muscles strong and helps joints remain flexible and supple.

Exercise is also a good way to beat stress and helps many people cope with anxiety and depression, and to sleep better.

What sort of exercise is best?

The best sort of exercise is the kind that requires stamina, like walking, swimming, running or cycling, rather than muscle-building exercise such as weight-lifting. Any exercise that makes you slightly breathless and makes your heart beat faster is beneficial to your heart.

Make sure you choose an exercise that you enjoy – that way you'll be far more likely to stick with it.

> **Those who do not exercise regularly are more than twice as likely to have a heart attack than those who do**

How much and how often?

The Government currently recommends that if you take no exercise at all then you should aim for 30 minutes of moderately vigorous exercise once a week. This should then be built up to 30 minutes a day most days of the week, and finally should include 20-30 minutes of vigorous exercise two or three times a week.

Sounds like a lot? If you haven't taken any exercise for a long time, start by finding more energetic ways of carrying out your everyday activities – walk to work, use the stairs or cycle to the shops. Build up your exercise gradually so that you get out of breath but not to the point of sprains or muscle strain!

Getting fit and staying fit means taking exercise regularly – unfortunately you can't store fitness!

- The above information is from the Coronary Prevention Group's web site which can be found at www.healthnet.org.uk

© Healthnet – 2002

Modes of travel to school

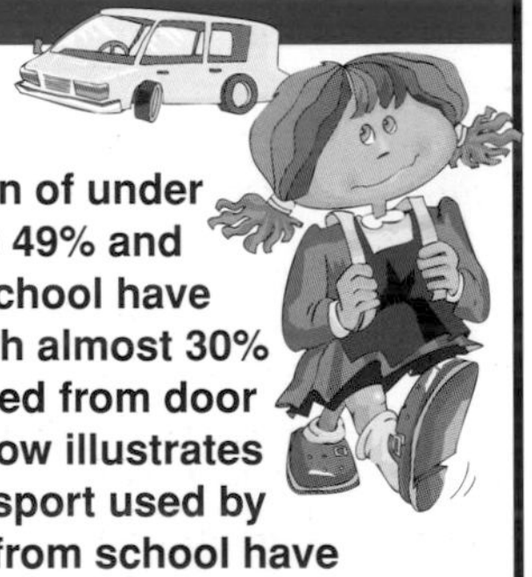

Active transportation, particularly to and from school, has decreased dramatically over recent decades. Between 1986 and 1996, the proportion of under 17-year-olds walking to schools fell from 59% to 49% and only 1% now cycle to school.[1] Car journeys to school have doubled in the last 20 years with almost 30% of pupils now being ferried from door to door.[1] The graph below illustrates how the modes of transport used by pupils to travel to and from school have changed between 1986 and 1996.[1]

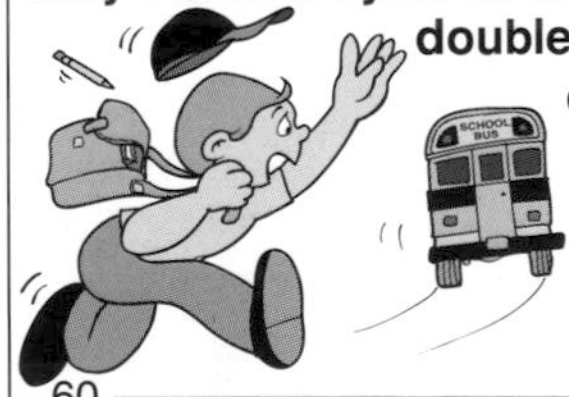

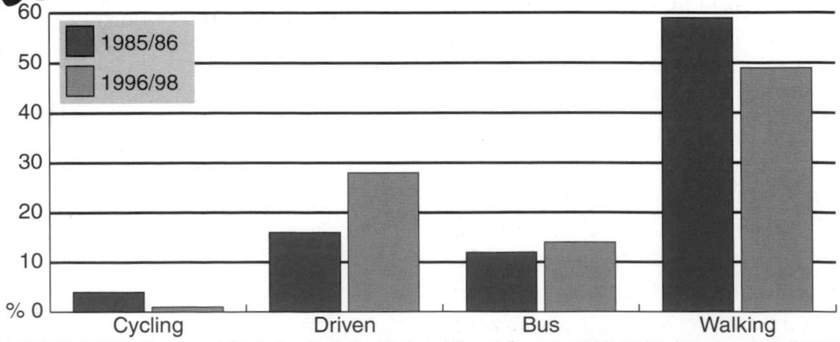

Legend: ■ 1985/86 ■ 1996/98

Bar chart (y-axis % from 0 to 60):
- Cycling: 1985/86 ≈ 4, 1996/98 ≈ 1
- Driven: 1985/86 ≈ 16, 1996/98 ≈ 28
- Bus: 1985/86 ≈ 12, 1996/98 ≈ 14
- Walking: 1985/86 ≈ 59, 1996/98 ≈ 49

1 DETR (1999). *Transport Statistics Bulletin*, National Travel Survey 1996-98 Update. London: DETR.

Source: Couch Kids - the growing epidemic – British Heart Foundation

Physical activity

Information from www.mindbodysoul.gov.uk

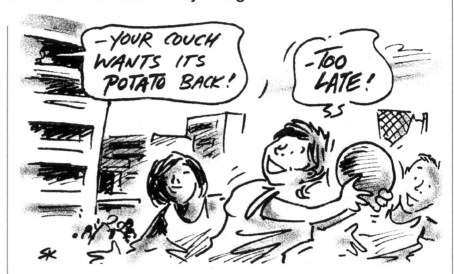

The good news is you don't have to be good at sport to be active. Small changes to your everyday routine, such as walking or cycling to school, increase your activity and help you to feel and look good. Activities like dancing and roller-blading are also a great way of increasing your activity and having fun at the same time!

As well as having fun, taking part in physical activity is a great way to:

- reduce boredom
- meet up with your mates and also meet new people
- unwind from your studies and relieve stress and tension.

And there are also lots of benefits to your health:

- weight control
- helping you to breathe more easily, which is especially important if you have asthma
- building stronger bones.

How much should I do?

Most young people of school age are physically active for about half an hour a day, most days of the week. This may sound good, but it's not enough to get the full health benefit. Ideally, you should be aiming for one hour of moderate intensity activity each day.

Moderate intensity activity makes you feel warm and breathe more heavily than usual. More vigorous activity is fine as long as you feel okay and still able to talk. This is known as your comfort zone. If you are unable to do this, you are probably working at too high an intensity. Check out your comfort zone.

You don't have to do one hour of activity all in one go. You can build up over the day – for example, 10 minutes walking to school, 20 minutes basketball at lunchtime, 10 minutes walking home from school and 20 minutes dancing around your room to your favourite tunes! Every little bit counts, but try to include some activity that is non-stop for 10-15 minutes – this would really help your heart health.

Warming up

For moderate to vigorous activities, you need to prepare your body for action. Your warm-up can be changed for different activities, but should include:

Activities that gradually raise the pulse

- Start with some gentle activity to gradually increase your heart rate. This ensures that the body is prepared gradually for the demands being made on it. Activities may include walking, gentle jogging, or cycling in a low gear.

Activities to mobilise the joints

- Mobility exercises involve slow, controlled movements of the muscles around those joints that will be used in the activity. For example, shoulder rotations, side bends and knee lifts.
- These should be performed with control, avoiding rapid flinging actions. Stand in a comfortable position, with knees slightly bent and feet apart and repeat each movement 6 to 8 times.

Stretching

- It is important to stretch the main muscle groups to be used in the activity for 6-10 seconds. For example, if the activity mainly involves leg work, stretches for the major leg muscles – the calves, quadriceps, hamstrings and groin – are required.

Cooling down

A cool-down after any moderate to vigorous physical activity will help to reduce the stiffness you sometimes get after activity. In the same way that the intensity of activity is gradually increased in the warm-up, it should be gradually decreased in the cool-down. The main types of activity that should be included are:

Activities to decrease the pulse rate

- One of the most effective cool-down activities is walking. Start with power walking, move through race walking and brisk walking and end with gentle walking.

Stretching

- A cool-down should include stretches for the muscle groups used in the activity. Stretches carried out in the warm-up can be repeated, but should be held for a minimum of 10-20 seconds and up to 60 seconds, where comfortable.

■ The above information is from the web site www.mindbodysoul.gov.uk

Fitness at college

Moving into higher education introduces you to a whole new range of leisure opportunities that you might never have thought about before. It's a chance to try out all kinds of different activities, usually for free or at very low cost. So what have you got to lose?

So many options

Most colleges have a gym, swimming pool or sports ground, and various classes and clubs to try out. If you are the sort of person who likes a bit of competition then you might have difficulty choosing between football, squash, basketball, rugby, netball, tennis, hockey, cricket, badminton, water polo, athletics and volleyball.

In the gym you can try your hand at ju jitsu, kickboxing, and akido, different kinds of aerobics, step workouts or body conditioning. If you want to tone up you can also try weight training, classes like 'Tums and Bums', boxercise, or circuit training.

Even if you don't think of yourself as the traditional sporty type, there are many other ways to get fit and stay healthy, including tai chi, women's self defence, yoga and the martial arts. Those who crave more adventure can get their adrenaline fixes by going out rock climbing, orienteering, horse riding, scuba diving, hang gliding, potholing, skiing, canoeing, parachuting, hiking and hot air ballooning. If you haven't seen anything that takes your fancy yet then it's relatively easy to get a few people together and start a club of your own.

Why bother?

But why should anybody bother getting all hot and sweaty when they could be at home nice and comfy watching daytime television or out drinking subsidised lager in the union bar all night? The good news is that

Even if you don't think of yourself as the traditional sporty type, there are many other ways to get fit

By Karla Fitzhugh

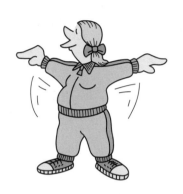

you only need to take two or three hours out of this thrilling weekly schedule to get all the benefits – and, let's face it, reruns of Ironside and Columbo will have lost their sparkle long before the end of the first term, and it's only a matter of time before Richard and Judy start getting on your nerves too.

Boosting your fitness levels will give you more energy and help you sleep better. Feeling like you are getting into shape also gives you a confidence boost. Regular exercise is a great stress buster, which is good to remember at exam time, and can even help relieve the symptoms of mild depression. Looking even further ahead, it can make a useful contribution to a CV when you are looking for work after graduation, so it might even give you the edge in landing your dream job. Employers value skills like teamwork, self-discipline and coping well with responsibility.

Keeping fit is also an easy way to make new friends, and lots of clubs organise social outings and parties, or just meet up regularly for drinks. And, of course, a fit body is an attractive body – which might well be a factor in meeting that special someone . . .

■ The above information is from YouthNet's web site which can be found at www.thesite.org

© TheSite.org

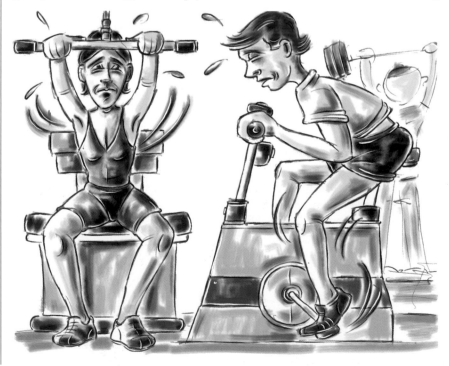

Personal trainer

**Ever thought about having a personal trainer?
Jonathan Richards takes a closer look**

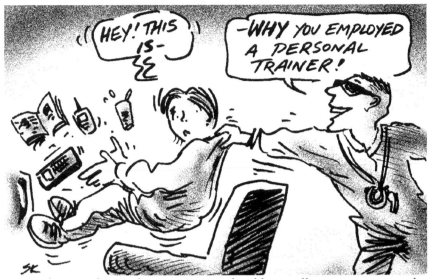

It used to be the case that anyone with a personal trainer was either a Hollywood film star or a nutter – the kind of person with far too much time and money on their hands and an unhealthy obsession for a butt like J-Lo's.

Why else pay £80 an hour for someone to yell at you while you're doing circuits in the gym or pounding your local park in the pissing rain when you'd much rather be at home watching telly? With over 5000 instructors in the UK, though, more and more people are using personal trainers. So what's it all about? And do they really work?

'It's not just about fitness,' says John Roberts, Company Director of Matt Roberts Training, who looks after the likes of Robbie Williams and Gucci Boss Tom Ford. 'You'll also find that training properly improves your posture, your outlook on life and even your relationships.'

Sounds expensive . . .

'It can be,' says Kenny Grieves, who runs Lancashire-based Evolution Personal Training, 'but you always have options. A top London professional can be £100 an hour but if you look around, certainly regionally, you can find a good trainer for £15 an hour. That means a one-on-one session and if that's still too pricey two or three of you can train together and share the cost.'

So how can I find a personal trainer?

There are two main options: a qualified trainer who visits you at home bringing basic equipment (like Kenny), or someone attached to a gym.

The best 'Home' trainers usually operate by referral from satisfied clients, while if you want a gym-based instructor it's better to aim for the bigger franchises – places like Fitness First and Holmes Place. These ensure qualified, capable trainers,

essential in an industry where anyone can operate even without professional qualifications.

So how do I avoid the cowboys?

Because personal training is so new there is no industry-wide body or specific qualification. However, Kenny suggests looking for WABA (World Amateur Bodybuilding Association) or EFBB (English Federation of Bodybuilders) accredited trainers. 'These are two of the main governing bodies and mean an instructor will be fully trained. In the case of WABA – the qualification I have – you have a residential course with two written exams, an oral and a practical, all pretty much to the standard of A-level Biology.'

As well as qualifications, a good trainer 'should also be more like a friend,' says John Roberts. 'You

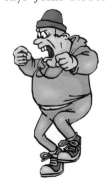

should actually start enjoying the sessions.'

Most important of all, a good trainer will thoroughly assess your fitness (blood pressure, heart rate, cardiovascular fitness etc.) and your objectives before devising you a set routine.

They should also:

- Change your training plan every 8-12 weeks (these are called MESO cycles and ensure your body is constantly working – or under Progressive Overload as the pros call it).
- Regularly test your overall fitness.
- Advise you on diet and nutrition.
- Encourage you to meet at least twice a week (after four days' inactivity you start to lose any fitness and muscle you gained).
- Place emphasis on both aerobic and bodybuilding exercises.

So is it really worth it?

If you can afford it, definitely. By using a personal trainer you'll progress 3-4 times faster, while having a pro on hand means you'll never get bored thanks to a constantly changing programme of exercises.

- The above information is from YouthNet's web site which can be found at www.thesite.org

Fitness the easy(er) way

You spend every waking moment snow boarding, entering karate competitions, skiing and sprinting round mazes, but you're still completely unfit. Maybe it's time to unplug the games console, leave Lara Croft at home and enter the real world! Advice by Karla Fitzhugh

You can have a healthy bod in the short space of about six weeks if you start some regular moderate exercise. It doesn't have to be painful or gruelling – and who knows, it might even be fun.

What to do?

Before you start, decide what you really want to get out of it. Is it: increased stamina, a flatter tum, or bigger muscles?

You can then choose the right kind of activities to reach your targets. If you have any kind of health problem, or are so unfit you can't climb the stairs without feeling breathless, then always go and see your doctor first for a check-up and some advice.

It's easier to stick to a routine if you can find something you really enjoy doing, because you're less likely to get bored and give up halfway through.

Try to get a friend to join you so that you can encourage each other to keep on going.

Doing it

Start your exercise regime gently, and slowly build up the time and effort that you put into it. Many fitness experts suggest that you begin with three 30-minute sessions per week.

Anything that gives you a continuous cardiovascular workout is suitable, including: jogging, swimming, rowing, cycling – and non-stop dancing!

You should be aiming to raise a slight sweat or need to breathe more deeply than you do at rest. Stop straight away if you begin to feel dizzy, wheezy or ill.

It's also really important to make sure you have the right equipment, such as comfortable kit and pair of trainers. If you are using a gym, get a proper induction and learn how to use the equipment safely.

Remember to warm up and warm down fully, and above all enjoy yourself!

■ The above information is from YouthNet's web site which can be found at www.thesite.org

© TheSite.org

The health benefits

The health benefits of regular physical activity are many. At least 30 minutes of moderate physical activity, for example brisk walking, is enough to bring many of these effects. However, by increasing the level of activity, the benefits will also increase.

Regular physical activity

■ reduces the risk of dying prematurely
■ reduces the risk of dying from heart disease or stroke, which are responsible for one-third of all deaths
■ reduces the risk of developing heart disease or colon cancer by up to 50%
■ reduces the risk of developing type II diabetes 50 %
■ helps to prevent/reduce hypertension, which affects one-fifth of the world's adult population
■ helps to prevent/reduce osteoporosis, reducing the risk of hip fracture by up to 50% in women
■ reduces the risk of developing lower back pain
■ promotes psychological well-being, reduces stress, anxiety and feelings of depression and loneliness
■ helps prevent or control risky behaviours, especially among children and young people, like tobacco, alcohol or other substance use, unhealthy diet or violence
■ helps control weight and lower the risk of becoming obese by 50% compared to people with sedentary lifestyles

■ helps build and maintain healthy bones, muscles, and joints and makes people with chronic, disabling conditions improve their stamina
■ can help in the management of painful conditions, like back pain or knee pain

We all know that physical activity – taking a walk, riding a bike, dancing or playing – simply makes you feel better. But regular physical activity brings about many other benefits. It not only has the potential to improve and maintain good health, but it can also bring with it important social and economic benefits.

Regular physical activity benefits communities and economies in terms of reduced healthcare costs, increased productivity, better performing schools, lower worker absenteeism and turnover, increased productivity and increased participation in sports and recreational activities.

In many countries, a significant proportion of health spending is due to costs related to lack of physical activity and obesity. Promoting physical activity can be a highly cost-effective and sustainable public health intervention.

■ The above information is from the World Health Organization's web site which can be found at www.who.int

© 2002 WHO/OMS

A guide to healthy socialising and exercise

Exercise for energy

You probably think you are fit or at least as fit as you need to be. But do you find you just haven't the energy to do the things you enjoy like socialising after the office, playing with the children, going for walks or doing the garden?

Just imagine a life where you could tap into enough energy to tackle a stressful job, cope with a demanding family and still have enough left over for yourself. If this seems like an impossible dream, it's time to get on the move. Regular exercise doesn't have to be boring, time consuming or expensive.

Choose the right class and you will feel less tired, increase your energy and achieve a more toned body. It also improves the function of your heart and lungs and strengthens your muscles to give you more stamina.

Exercise keeps your joints mobile and increases your circulation which makes your skin look healthier and you look younger. Above all it produces a wonderful feeling of well-being which makes you better able to deal with whatever life throws at you!

The benefits of exercise

Once you start to exercise regularly you will feel more confident and relaxed. Stress and tension will become things of the past. Exercise classes are exhilarating and friendly and you will soon start to feel better mentally and physically.

New-found energy increases self-confidence, and can also be a springboard to becoming involved in other new sports such as cycling, climbing, swimming, ice skating or rollerblading! Other benefits of exercise include:

■ *A decrease in resting heart rate*: Exercise strengthens your heart so it doesn't need to beat as often to pump blood through your body. Doing everyday activities such as mowing the lawn or running up the stairs can be completed with less stress on your heart.

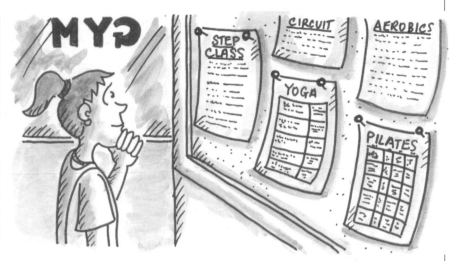

■ *A drop in blood pressure*
If your blood pressure is slightly above normal, regular exercise can help to bring it down.

■ *Soaring energy levels*
You'll be amazed – those tough days at work and those demanding times with the children or family won't wear you out so much. Whether it be sailing, playing a game of tennis or climbing a mountain, you will also have much more energy to devote to the activities you enjoy doing he most.

■ *Lower risk of heart disease*
By reducing stress, blood pressure and cholesterol while increasing the strength and efficiency of the heart, regular low impact exercise can help reduce the risk of coronary heart disease.

■ *A leaner more toned body*
Regular exercise helps to speed up your metabolism, which means you increase the rate of energy burned during and after exercise, which helps to decrease body fat.

Exercise keeps your joints mobile and increases your circulation which makes your skin look healthier and you look younger

---

Keep motivated

The hardest thing with exercise can be keeping motivated and sticking to it. Here are some tips to keep you going:

■ Set yourself realistic goals. Work out what you want to achieve and go for it.

■ Choose an activity you will enjoy, is sociable and will not become boring.

■ Reward yourself for progress but not with chocolate! What about a relaxing body treat such as an aromatherapy message, a neck and shoulder massage or a manicure?

■ Going to classes with a friend often helps to keep you going. Verbal encouragement and reinforcement are great sources of confidence.

Exercise develops strength, stamina and flexibility – the best investment you can make for your future. You will be able to play sport with your children and grandchildren as well as running for the train.

Healthy muscles give your body shape and tone while flexibility will keep you mobile as you age. Strong muscles mean good support for your skeleton and therefore good posture.

■ The above information is an extract from *A guide to healthy socialising and exercise*, produced by the Fitness League. See page 41 for their address details.

© *The Fitness League*

Exercise your way to a long and healthy life

Information from the Fitness Industry Association

Is your six-pack looking more like a keg or your love handles beginning to resemble wing mirrors? We know you've heard it all before and you might not be worried about a bit of extra flesh here and there, but do you realise the damage your sedentary lifestyle could be doing to your overall health?

While many people associate exercise with looking good, the benefits of exercise aren't directly linked with your overall body shape. However, the body does need exercise to maintain itself for its daily duties and your physical well-being can determine the long-term quality of your life.

For instance: the body is held together by a network of tissues and more than 600 muscles. Weakened muscles cannot support a heavy skeleton and so your posture will ultimately suffer. Also the more active muscle you have, the higher your metabolic rate and the more fat you will burn, even in your sleep!

The heart is one big muscle, which beats an incredible 100,000 times a day and is responsible for pumping blood around the body. Activity exercises the heart, making it beat faster and strengthening it in a similar manner to other muscles. Studies show that regular exercise can reduce the risk of heart attack or stroke by almost a half.

As your breathing increases during exercise your lungs further expand and contract, allowing more oxygen to infiltrate the bloodstream, and toxic gases to be exhaled with greater proficiency.

Exercise could improve your looks too! Your skin may look clearer and younger, as more toxins are passed out of the body during activity, and facial muscles also receive a toning and firming 'workout'.

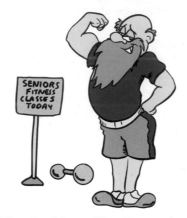

Physical benefits of exercise

- Helps to control blood pressure and improves blood circulation
- Reduces the risk of heart disease and strokes
- Improves lung function
- Aids weight control
- Improves posture
- Helps to make bones stronger, reducing the risk of osteoporosis (brittle bone disease)
- Strengthens and tones muscles
- Relieves menstrual problems, pre-menstrual syndrome and constipation
- Can slow the ageing process

Mental benefits of exercise

- Provides a 'feel good' factor
- Relieves depression and anxiety, reducing stress

- Improves self-awareness, self-confidence and self-esteem
- Increases emotional stimulation, mental stimulation and improves memory in the elderly

So we've convinced you that it's time to take action, but finding a suitable health club or fitness centre can be a daunting thought if you've never exercised before. What should you be looking for?

The first is to seek out a Fitness Industry Association (FIA) member's plaque. The FIA is the trade body representing the whole of the health and fitness sector, including more than 1,400 health clubs and fitness centres around the UK.

The FIA's main role is to promote excellence and best practice within the industry, and all FIA member clubs work towards a Code of Practice, a set of performance standards – so you can be sure you're in good hands right from the start.

The Code's health and safety guidelines mean that your best interests are at the forefront of their minds: consistent high standards mean they will do their utmost to keep the facilities in the best working order at all times.

Customer care is another important factor within the Code,

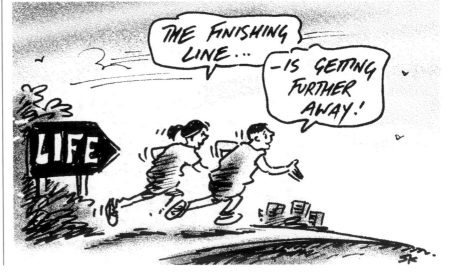

and you'll be made welcome in what is often thought of as an intimidating environment, by people who understand your needs. You'll be welcome, safe and well looked after.

In addition, the FIA and SPRITO (the industry's National Training Organisation) have recently launched a Register of Exercise Professionals. The register will form a comprehensive list of qualified fitness instructors throughout the UK, offering peace of mind to members of the public trusting their health and safety to exercise tutors.

The Fitness Industry Association also runs the fitness industry-acclaimed FLAME awards (Fitness Leadership And Management Excellence), which identify and applaud the very best in the business, further encouraging and promoting the delivery of high-quality customer care.

Committed to the improvement of public health and well-being, the FIA promotes regular exercise through national campaigns, such as Commit to Get Fit, Europe's largest fitness campaign, which attracts more participants than the London marathon! Now heading for its eleventh year, the summer campaign raises vital funds for its sponsor charity, so watch out for signs at your local health and fitness club or leisure centre.

Top tips to help you stick with it

It's always a good idea to find a centre close to home or work. If you've got the excuse of traffic jams or busy schedules it's all too easy to take the *mañana* approach.

Find a friend to exercise with. Not only will you have added encouragement and more fun, but you'll feel guilty about letting them down to take a night off.

Make time to exercise. Plan well ahead, setting dates to exercise in your diary, and book classes so you can't drop out.

Remember – exercise gives you more energy, so you'll feel less tired, will do things quicker and ultimately have more free time! Exercise also releases 'feel good' chemicals called endorphins, so you'll feel happier and less stressed after a good workout.

Take it slowly, and don't expect to keep up with the instructors. Getting through the doors is the biggest hurdle. If you can manage that you'll soon be on your way to a fitter, healthier, happier lifestyle.

One session a week is a success. The key is to commit to regular attendance (at whatever level). Higher frequency of visits will develop once you have a regular routine as a base.

Set yourself realistic goals and move the goal posts little by little every 6-8 weeks. However, you should start to feel results in less than a month.

If you can't get to the gym try taking the stairs during the day, it burns off 8.5 calories per minute. And walk short distances instead of driving, at a brisk pace you can burn off between 200-300 calories per hour, as well as exercising more than 250 muscles. Reward yourself with a sauna, jacuzzi or gentle swim after your workout.

Everyone needs to give in to temptation now and then, but by understanding and following the basic principles of healthy living, and making regular exercise a way of life, you could well increase the length of your life too. Try to follow the guidelines below whenever possible:
1. Avoid smoking
2. Drink alcohol in moderation
3. Eat a well-balanced diet
4. Keep your weight under control
5. Exercise regularly
6. Aim to reduce your stress levels
   Some facts courtesy of BUPA and the Leisure Corporation.
   © Fitness Industry Association

What is a healthy diet?

Information from the Obesity Resource and Information Centre (ORIC)

Food is an integral part of our everyday lives and should also provide much pleasure. The sayings 'moderation in all things' and 'variety is the spice of life' are surprisingly apt when it comes to talking about a healthy balanced diet.

We all recognise that choosing to eat the right foods can make an important contribution to good health, but with the vast range of fresh and processed foods now available and the immense media coverage of food and health issues, many people find it increasingly difficult to select the foods which together provide a diet for optimum health.

A balanced diet provides the energy (calories) and nutrients we need, not just to survive but also to stay fit and healthy. Food is made up of macronutrients (protein, fat, carbohydrate and alcohol) which are essential for growth, body maintenance and provide energy, and micronutrients (vitamins, minerals and trace elements) which are only needed in very small amounts but are essential to regulate the body's chemical processes and functions. Some minerals also have a structural role, for example calcium in bones and teeth. Fruit, vegetables, pulses and whole grains also contain bio-active compounds known as 'phytochemicals' which appear to have beneficial effects on health.

The word 'diet' is often used to refer to a special eating pattern, especially for someone trying to lose weight, but it more correctly describes what a person usually eats and drinks. If an individual's usual diet does not meet his or her nutritional needs he or she will eventually become ill. For example, a low iron intake will lead to anaemia which causes tiredness, weakness and ultimately death. A diet will also be poorly balanced if the foods are not consumed in healthy proportions. For example, the diet may contain too many high fat foods or too few fruits and vegetables. Unbalanced diets increase the risk of long-term health problems, such as heart disease, cancer, obesity, tooth decay, gall stones and osteoporosis.

Choosing a healthy balanced diet

In 1997 the Government produced a set of guidelines for a healthy diet. These are:

- Enjoy your food.
- Eat a variety of different foods.
- Eat the right amount to be a healthy weight.
- Eat plenty of foods rich in starch and fibre.
- Eat plenty of fruit and vegetables.
- Don't eat too many foods that contain a lot of fat.
- Don't have sugary foods and drinks too often.
- If you drink alcohol, drink sensibly.

In June 1999 the Government published the White Paper *Saving Lives: Our Healthier Nation* which is an action plan to tackle poor health. Action to provide a healthier diet (e.g. plenty of fruit, vegetables and cereals, and not too much fatty and salty food) for all is one of the key recommendations of the paper, as is assisting people to maintain appropriate body weights for their physique.

The Health Education Authority 'Balance of Good Health' depicts these guidelines in terms of five different groups of foods, showing the proportions for a healthy balanced diet.

Breads, other cereals and potatoes – which should form the basis of every meal.

Fruit and vegetables – aim for at least five portions every day.

Milk and dairy foods – eat or drink a moderate amount of these foods, about two to three servings per day.

Meat, fish and alternatives – eat moderate amounts of these foods – about two servings per day.

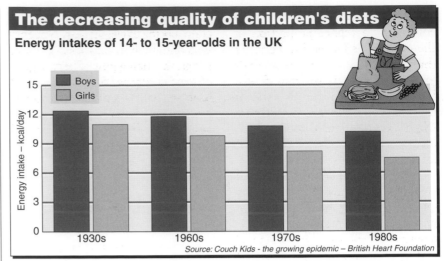

The decreasing quality of children's diets

Energy intakes of 14- to 15-year-olds in the UK

Source: Couch Kids - the growing epidemic – British Heart Foundation

Foods containing fat and foods containing sugar – in small amounts only.

Foods in each of the first four food groups are good sources of nutrients that the body needs for good health. Foods in the fifth group are high in fat and/or sugar and do not provide such wide variety of essential nutrients, but are high in energy (calories). A diet containing too many items from group five will provide excessive amounts of energy if it is also to include adequate protein and micronutrients. Although, in moderation these foods add extra choice and enjoyment to meals, for people trying to lose weight these foods should be reduced in order to decrease the total energy intake, without compromising the intake of essential nutrients.

Making sense of food labels

Nutrition information on food labels can help guide consumers towards healthy food choices. They can be used to check and compare similar products to see which are, for example, lower in fat or salt, or higher in fibre. Nutrition claims need to be assessed carefully. A 'low fat' claim means that the product should have no more than 3g of fat per 100g. 'Reduced fat' only indicates the product has less fat than the traditional variety (the guideline is 25% less). It may still be a high fat food. For example, reduced fat crisps may contain 30% less fat than traditional crisps, but still have around 20g of fat per 100g.

The following daily guideline intakes give a guide as to how much energy, fat, salt and fibre is recommended in a healthy diet for a man or woman of average size. Larger people, or those who are very physically active, will have higher energy needs, whilst smaller people, or those who lead very sedentary lives will have lower nutrient requirements. Using these guidelines the nutritional information on foods can be examined to see how food can fit into healthy diets.

Foods	Men	Women
Calories	2,500	2,000
Fat	95 g	70 g
Saturated Fat	30 g	20 g
Sugar	70 g	50 g
Fibre	20 g	16 g
Sodium (salt)	2.5g	2 g

An adequate intake of vitamins and minerals is also essential for a healthy diet. The recommended amounts for the general population are set out as part of the Government report on 'Dietary Reference Values.' Some nutritional labels on food products also mention one or more of the vitamins and minerals if the food item is a particularly rich source or if a nutritional claim is made with regard to the nutrient.

Dietary guidelines for the prevention of obesity

A healthy balanced diet plays an important role in the prevention of obesity. There is considerable evidence to suggest that the proportion of fat in the diet is important in determining the risk of obesity. Studies show that people consuming a higher proportion of their energy as fat tend to be fatter than people who obtain most of their energy from carbohydrate foods. Research studies have also shown that lean volunteers tend to eat more when they are offered foods which are higher in fat relative to low fat foods.

When the energy (calorie) input from food and drink matches energy output (through metabolism and physical activity) an individual is described as being in 'energy balance' and their weight will be stable. If energy input is greater than output they will no longer be in 'energy balance', the excess energy will be stored (mainly as fat) and they will begin to gain weight. Alternatively, decreasing energy input and/or increasing energy output will result in weight loss. To lose 1 lb (0.5 kg) of body fat requires an energy deficit of 3,500 calories (vice versa for gaining it).

There are a number of reasons why fat is particularly fattening:

- Fat adds taste and texture to food making it particularly palatable and moreish.

- Fat is very energy dense; that is, it contains more than twice as many calories per gram as protein and carbohydrate. This means that high fat foods contain more calories per mouthful than lower fat foods.

- Fat seems to promote a reduced sense of satiety or fullness compared to protein or carbohydrate-rich foods. The result is that more fat calories are eaten to get the same 'I've had enough to eat' feeling that comes from carbohydrate or protein-rich foods.

Put together this means that energy intake tends to be much higher on a high fat diet relative to a lower fat diet and hence weight gain is more likely. Furthermore, there is good evidence that by switching to a diet where some of the energy from fat is replaced by carbohydrate, it is possible to moderate energy intake and so help people to maintain their body weight.

Evidence also suggests that alcohol can increase energy intake thus potentially contributing to weight gain. Not only is alcohol high in calories (7 calories per gram – half a pint of beer or glass of wine contains 85 calories), but it is also usually drunk in addition to usual food intake, promotes storage of body fat, stimulated appetite and disinhibits voluntary restraint – all a lethal combination of over-indulgence!

Currently, the advice for both the prevention and treatment of obesity focuses on decreasing the amount of fat in the diet and increasing the intake of fruit and vegetables

---

In order to lose weight it is essential to decrease energy intake below an individual's energy needs. In this way the additional energy which is needed by the body is taken from the existing body fat stores. To lose one kilogram of fat requires an energy deficit of 7,000 calories. The recommended rate of weight loss is 0.5 to 1 kg per week. This requires an energy deficit of between 500 and 1,000 calories per day. This can best be achieved by reducing the amount of fat in the diet and also decreasing the amount of food eaten in general. The efficacy of any dietary plan can

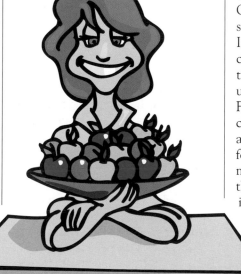

be enhanced by a gradual increase in the amount of physical activity.

Many people are often tempted to follow diets that are very low in calories and which promise rapid weight loss. Certainly, in the first week the weight loss in these diets can be extremely rapid but only a small proportion of the weight which is lost will be fat – much of it is fluid. Moreover, after losing weight many people quickly return to their former eating habits and weight is regained. This type of crash dieting does not help people to learn to adjust their eating habits to provide a diet which is sustainable in the long term, and can also lead to a loss of confidence in their ability to lose weight.

Making dietary changes

In order to reduce the risk of weight gain and/or to treat an existing weight problem it is necessary to make long-term changes in our eating habits. By their nature eating habits are long-established and therefore difficult to change. Some key aspects of any programme to change eating habits include motivation, confidence and support. Few people successfully change their eating habits because they are told to do so, in almost all cases the individual must want to change. Confidence to succeed can be enhanced by careful planning of any changes. Many people find it useful to keep a food diary to help them become more aware of what they eat, when and why. Some people may find that they benefit from professional support if they regularly eat to cope with anxiety and stress. Confidence can also be enhanced by setting moderate and realistic goals. It is much better to successfully change one aspect of the diet at a time, rather than trying to make unachievable wholesale changes. Finally, it is always easier to make changes with the support of family and friends. Currently, the advice for both the prevention and treatment of obesity focuses on decreasing the amount of fat in the diet and increasing the intake of fruit and vegetables. This eating plan can form the basis of a healthy diet for the whole family.

© *The Obesity Resource and Information Centre (ORIC)*

Food fitness

Lifestyle tips

Meet the Activaters
... they get more out of life by being active and eating a healthy diet. They are full of energy and enjoy good health.

Meet the Dolittles
... they avoid all forms of physical activity and their diet could be improved. That's why they are putting on weight.

Be active in your daily life
You don't have to be a sporty type to be an Activater. Going for a walk, doing the housework or carrying the shopping are all effective. Just putting a bit more effort into physical tasks and relying less on labour-saving devices is an excellent start.

Walking is one of the easiest ways of being more active. You don't have to buy special clothing or spend hours in the gym. Walking is free and it's something nearly everyone can do. Regular, brisk walking actually lowers the risk of heart disease.

If you've been more of a Dolittle than an Activater up to now, don't try to do too much all in one go. Take it step by step. Gradually build up your activity levels then keep up the good work – because staying fit means staying active.

Take pleasure in active leisure
Think about adding some activity to your leisure time. Your local parks and leisure centres will have plenty of activities to try: bowls, cricket, football, roller blading, swimming and lots more. See which one suits you best. Alternatively, try dancing, gardening or energetic DIY to keep you active.

Set realistic goals for yourself. Begin gradually and build up both the length and level of activity. Dolittles should start off with one or two 30-minute sessions a week. If 30 minutes in one go is difficult, try two 15-minute sessions.

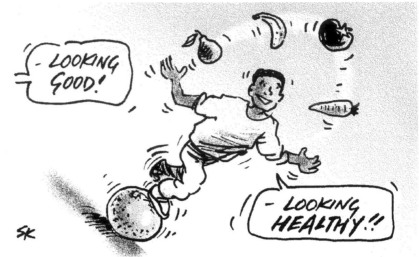

If you have a medical condition, or are recovering from illness, check with your doctor before you start.

For maximum health benefits Activaters should aim to build up to 30 minutes of moderate activity five times a week. That means moving about enough to make you feel warm and slightly out of breath. There's no need to push yourself too hard even if you think you are fit. You should never be too breathless to talk.

Vary your activities so that all your muscles get exercised. This will also reduce the risk of injury.

Aim for 5 fruit and veg a day
Fruit and vegetables are an excellent source of the vitamins, minerals and fibre we need to help maintain a healthy body and fight diseases. Yet most of us don't eat enough of them.

Try to eat at least five portions of fruit and vegetables each day. This may sound a lot but the good news is that a glass of orange juice, an apple, a small can of tomatoes or baked beans each counts as one portion.

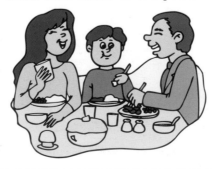

Potatoes don't count here although they are important in the diet for other reasons.

Different types of fruit and veg provide different nutrients in varying amounts, so choosing from a wide variety of them is best. With a bit of forward planning you will see that it's easy to meet the 5-a-day goal without having to make major changes to your eating habits.

Base meals on starchy foods
Starches, along with sugars, are known as carbohydrates. They are an important part of our diet because carbohydrate is the body's favourite fuel.

Make starchy foods (bread, potatoes, cereals, rice and pasta) the basis of your main meals. For example, have a bigger helping of pasta and a smaller helping of the sauce. Increasing the proportion of carbohydrate in our diet can actually help control weight. Eating starchy foods, especially wholegrain varieties, increases your fibre intake too.

Be careful to increase just the carbohydrates and not the fat in your diet. Limit how much fat such as butter, margarine, mayonnaise and creamy sauces you add to bread, pasta and other starchy foods. Choose boiled rather than fried rice and baked or boiled potatoes rather than roast or fried. Use semi-skimmed milk for mashed potatoes and less butter.

Snacks are also a useful source of carbohydrates and other nutrients, especially as you become more active. But remember to check out food labels to keep track of the fat content.

Check out more lower fat choices

Fat has twice as many calories as carbohydrate and protein – eating too much of it can easily lead to weight gain. But, some fat in the diet is essential for health.

Cutting down on fat doesn't have to mean totally changing your diet. Most people can do it by making a few small changes to everyday meals. Compare a Dolittle's meal with an Activater's meal – they are basically the same foods, but the fat content is quite different.

As most of us eat too much fat, the chances are that if you make more lower fat choices you are helping your health. But remember: children under five should not follow a low fat diet. At that age they need more energy from fat for healthy growth and development.

Grams of fat	
Mr Dolittle's Meal	
Rump Steak, grilled (with fat)	18.8
Chips	15.0
Peas (boiled)	0.3
Mushrooms (fried)	8.1
Yogurt (creamy)	6.0
Total fat (grams)	**48.2**
Total Energy (kcal)	**941**

Mr Activater's Meal	
Rump Steak, grilled (without fat)	9.3
Baked (jacket) potato	0.4
with 2 tsp low fat spread	4.5
Peas (boiled)	0.3
Mushrooms (grilled)	0.2
Yogurt (low fat)	1.1
Total fat (grams)	**15.8**
Total Energy (kcal)	**650**

■ The above information is an extract from the Food and Drink Federation's foodfitness campaign web site which can be found at www.foodfitness.org.uk

© Food and Drink Federation

Sensible eating

Information from Absolute Fitness

When it comes to eating, sensible doesn't have to equal boring, and a healthy, balanced diet doesn't mean living like a monk. A little bit of what you like is part of a balanced diet; many people who give up trying to change their eating habits do so because they have denied themselves everything they like. Life is for living, so if you want some chocolate, have some! Just don't eat several bars in one go!

Eating healthily is about a lifestyle change – not a short-term crash diet. Crash diets do not work!! Sensible eating patterns combined with regular exercise will help you remain fit and healthy, and also to lose weight if that is your goal. Once you are in the habit of eating well and exercising, it really does become part of everyday life.

You need to eat a balance of proteins, carbohydrates, fruit, vegetables, pulses and grains. The daily requirements of each food group can be put together to create a food pyramid, with what you need most of at the base and the smallest amount forming the pinnacle. Carbohydrates form the base, followed by fruit and veg, then dairy produce, meat and

fish, and finally fat. The percentages you should be roughly aiming for in your daily diet are:

Healthy balance	
Carbohydrates	40%
Vegetables	17.5%
Fruit	17.5%
Dairy products	10%
Meat/fish/pulses	10%
Fats/oils	%

When it comes to maintaining energy levels throughout the day, eating the right amounts at the right time is the most important factor – the cliché is to 'breakfast like a king, lunch like a prince, and dine like a pauper'. Unfortunately most of us get it the wrong way round – no time for breakfast, grab a bit of lunch, and eat a feast at night.

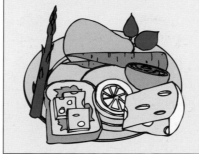

Eating at the wrong times, and skipping meals altogether, leads to low blood sugar levels (hypoglycaemia). This results in tiredness, irritability, a lack of co-ordination, headaches, and a sudden urge to eat half a pound of chocolate!

Snacking on chocolate or sweets sends the blood sugar soaring (hyperglycaemia), resulting in the release of a large dose of insulin, designed to help the body disperse excess sugar. But the body always overcompensates – sending blood sugar levels too low, and putting you back where you started: hungry, tired, and irritable.

So use your common sense when deciding what to eat and when – 10 pints of lager and a curry before bedtime is not going to do your waistline any favours. Arm yourself with a little knowledge, and just concentrate on getting it right every day – before you know it you won't even have to think about it.

■ The above information is from the Absolute Fitness web site: www.absolutefitness.co.uk

© Absolute Fitness

Guidelines for a healthier diet

Information from the Institute of Food Research

Eat a wide variety of different foods

No food needs to be totally excluded from your diet – except occasionally for special medical reasons. Try to eat foods from each of the four main groups (starchy foods, dairy products, meat and fish, fruit and vegetables) each day and vary these over the week. If you don't eat meat and/or fish, pay particular attention to finding sensible alternatives.

Eat the right amount to be a healthy weight

Try to fill up on low fat foods or those with less calories, like starchy foods, fruit or vegetables.

Eat plenty of fruit and vegetables

Try to consume at least five portions of fruits and vegetables per day. Potatoes are a useful source of several essential nutrients but don't count them as one of your vegetable servings. Pile your plate with colour; the fruits and vegetables with coloured flesh appear to be important in the protective quality of these foods.

Eat plenty of foods rich in starch and fibre

Try to base most of your meals around foods that are rich in starch and fibre (bread, pasta, rice, breakfast cereals, potatoes, etc.). These are versatile and usually cheap. Go continental and serve bread with every meal. Increasing your intake of starchy foods will also lead to a reduction in your fat intake.

Try to limit fat intake

We must have some fat in our diets because they are needed to absorb fat soluble vitamins or are essential to our health. However, too much fat in the diet, along with other factors such as smoking and lack of

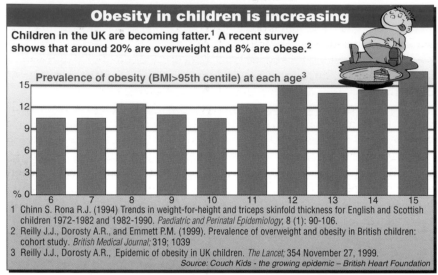

Obesity in children is increasing

Children in the UK are becoming fatter.[1] A recent survey shows that around 20% are overweight and 8% are obese.[2]

Prevalence of obesity (BMI>95th centile) at each age[3]

1 Chinn S. Rona R.J. (1994) Trends in weight-for-height and triceps skinfold thickness for English and Scottish children 1972-1982 and 1982-1990. *Paediatric and Perinatal Epidemiology;* 8 (1): 90-106.
2 Reilly J.J., Dorosty A.R., and Emmett P.M. (1999). Prevalence of overweight and obesity in British children: cohort study. *British Medical Journal;* 319; 1039
3 Reilly J.J., Dorosty A.R., Epidemic of obesity in UK children. *The Lancet;* 354 November 27, 1999.
Source: Couch Kids - the growing epidemic – British Heart Foundation

exercise, increases the risk of a heart attack or stroke. In this country we eat much more fat than we need and the UK has one of the highest incidences of heart disease in the world.

■ Choose low fat dairy products and lean cuts of meat. Try grilling or baking instead of frying or roasting, and don't add fat during cooking. If you do use a cooking fat, try one that is low in saturated fats. Remember that fat has twice as many calories as the same weight of carbohydrate or protein.

■ Children under five are growing rapidly, so cutting down their fat intake too much may mean they won't be getting enough energy. Don't cut down on fat for children under two.

Choose fruit or bread rather than chocolate or sweets

Eating sugary foods is the main cause of tooth decay. Sugars contain calories and no other nutrients.

Look after the vitamins and minerals in your food

Store foods properly and eat them as fresh as possible. Overcooking vegetables and boiling them in too much water will destroy much of

their nutritive value. Try steaming, pressure cooking or microwave cooking.

If you drink, keep within sensible limits

It is recommended that men should drink less than 21 units of alcohol a week, and women less than 14 (1 unit is half a pint of average beer or lager, a glass of wine or a pub measure of spirits). Make your drinks last longer by taking smaller sips or adding a mixer or mineral water. If you want to drink more try the low alcohol or alcohol free drinks now available.

Taste your food before adding salt

On average we eat about 13 grams (2 teaspoons) of salt a day, but we only need about 3 grams ($^1/_2$ teaspoon). Too much salt can lead to high blood pressure. Most of the salt is added during food manufacturing, so choose unsalted foods and don't add salt during cooking.

Based on information from the Health Education Authority and the World Health Organization.

■ The above information is from the Institute of Food Research's web site: www.ifr.bbsrc.ac.uk

© *Institute of Food Research*

Have a banana

In the US, fast-food chains are being sued by overweight customers. Here, too, obesity is a growing problem. Helen Carter reports on a Liverpool scheme to promote healthier eating among children

The statistics are alarming: as many as one in 10 children in Britain aged under four is obese, while one in five adults is dangerously overweight. Obesity costs the NHS an estimated £500m a year and it costs the economy £2bn through sickness and premature deaths (of which there are around 31,000 a year).

Rates of obesity among children have doubled in the past 20 years and a forum of education and health professionals heard earlier this year that a generation of children is eating itself sick with a diet high in fat and salt-saturated food. Unless urgent action is taken to correct the diets of young people, the experts gathered at the Royal College of Paediatrics and Child Health conference in London warned, young people risk being less healthy than those brought up during post-war rationing. Relatively sedentary lifestyles have compounded the problems.

There is also evidence that type two diabetes is emerging in severely overweight teenagers, a condition that had previously only ever been recorded in adults over 40.

Research from the Institute of Child Health found that two-thirds of pre-school children have a poor diet that is heavily reliant on white bread, chips, crisps and sweets.

The backlash against junk food has already begun in America, with a $50m lawsuit being launched against a US food manufacturer after it suddenly doubled the fat content of a supposedly healthy snack. The lawsuit claims emotional distress and nutritional damage has been caused by the food company's product.

So what is being done in schools to counter the crisis in eating habits? In Liverpool, a partnership involving the city council, health professionals, schools and the university has been devised to combat poor eating habits and prevent problems in future generations.

> **Research from the Institute of Child Health found that two-thirds of pre-school children have a poor diet that is heavily reliant on white bread, chips, crisps and sweets**

Part of the programme, known as Sportlinx, consists of a series of after-school and breakfast clubs specifically centred around nutrition. A pilot programme began earlier this year and taster sessions have also taken place at 25 schools across the city.

The after-school ventures consist of food, cookery and nutrition clubs that have been developed for primary school children at key stage 2 (year 5 or 6). They aim to increase the children's awareness of practical cooking skills and the importance of healthy eating.

The club delivers fun, interactive sessions covering nutrition and practical cookery. The children take their efforts home to their families. It begins with a food intake and lunchbox questionnaire to assess the children's eating habits and in-corporates balancing their diet, carbohydrates, fat, protein and fibre and pulses.

Before the course began, nine out of 10 of the children who took part in the after-school nutrition clubs had never heard of couscous. But they all learned how to make simple and healthy recipes such as fresh fruit kebabs with a yoghurt dip, mixed vegetable couscous, chicken and sweetcorn pasta, smoked mackerel on crispbread and fruity wholemeal and oat muffins.

St Christopher's RC primary school in Speke is one of the pilot schools that also runs a breakfast club in the morning. It is on the edge of the city on a large council estate close to Liverpool John Lennon Airport – the control tower is visible from the first floor and there is an audible hum of planes taking off. The school, which this year celebrates its 50th anniversary, is in an education action zone.

Part of the problem is that the estate is not served by any major supermarkets, which makes it difficult when trying to encourage people to eat healthily, as fresh fruit is not immediately accessible.

At the after-school nutrition club, a group of 10- and 11-year-olds were chopping up brightly coloured pieces of fruit to make kebabs. They were all wearing aprons emblazoned with Funky Food Club – the name they had chosen among themselves.

Joanna Clayton and Daniel Bird, both 11, casually munched on red apples after they had finished preparing the fruit kebabs. Daniel said: 'It has given us a chance to learn about what is healthy and how to cook things more healthily. I used to eat a lot of sweets and chocolate and crisps, but since I came to the Funky Food Club I have learnt how bad they are for you and how important it is to eat five portions of fruit a day.' He says his mum has now

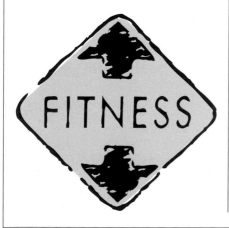

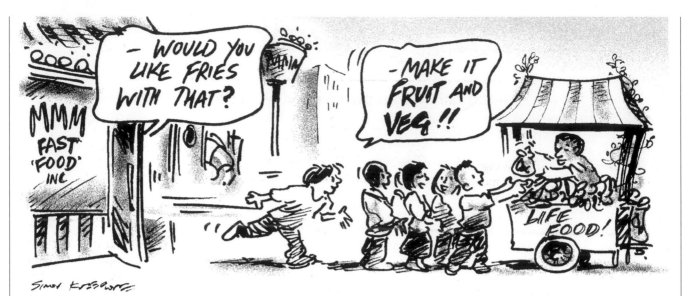

started to buy more fruit instead of junk food.

Joanne says she now likes to eat carrots (laced with a little salt), grapes and strawberries. 'My mum and dad always want to try the things I have brought home and they always look forward to seeing what I am going to bring home,' she says. 'My dad works late and we have always eaten the food before he gets home.'

Dr Brian Johnson, a nutritionist with South Liverpool Primary Care Trust, who helped to devise the programme, says the children fill in a pre-club evaluation questionnaire about their eating habits. 'When we collect the data we are getting an idea of their eating habits, which are likely to include too many fatty and sugary foods, and we are trying to encourage them to eat more starchy foods,' he says.

'The key to giving them information is to make it relevant to them – we can't just talk to them about health. They have got to taste things they have never tasted before. When we were using couscous, it was the first time that nine out of 10 of the kids had the opportunity to taste it.

'We are showing them that healthy food can taste OK – it doesn't have to be like sawdust.'

He says they start by asking what their favourite foods are. 'We are saying that burgers, chips and chocolate bars are not all bad, but they have to be balanced with healthy things. We introduce them to kiwi fruit, sharon fruit, passion fruit and mango, which are not readily available on this estate, as it doesn't have a big supermarket.

'I always say to people that there is no quicker food than eating an apple. It is the ultimate convenience food; you don't even have to unwrap it.'

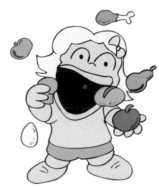

Eleven-year-old Sarah Kirwin admitted that she was not aware of what foods were healthy before the after-school nutrition club began. 'I would not have eaten any fruits and I didn't think that fish was healthy,' she said. 'Before, I used to eat chicken, ham, crisps and chocolate – but I have learnt how bad it is for you.

'I have been surprised by the colours and textures of the fruit. I had not tried things like mango and kiwi fruit. I am trying to encourage my mum to buy more fruit and vegetables and I feel healthier in

---

'We are showing them that healthy food can taste OK – it doesn't have to be like sawdust'

---

myself. When my mum went to put some chips on I asked her to do something else instead because I didn't want any.'

Her friend Nicola Seddon, also 11, said: 'I used to sit around watching television after school but now I am more active, playing football and athletics and playing on a trampoline. Once we were going to have something from the chippy for tea but I brought home what I had made at the Funky Food Club and we had that instead, and my family didn't mind.'

Hazel Cheung, a home economist at John Moores University in Liverpool, who is teaching the children, says the key is to get children interested in eating healthily and developing basic cooking skills.

'We need to move away from a McDonald's culture,' Cheung says. 'We are trying to promote healthy eating as being fun and to develop an interest in food that will produce healthier kids and reduce diabetes.

'Good nutrition needs to start from birth, really. Health professionals are quite distraught and shocked that teenagers nowadays can't cook. Most people think healthy eating involves vegetarians, weird people or posh people and we are trying to make it fun. We are saying there is nothing wrong with the occasional fast food – we are not food police. We are trying to be realistic, promoting more fruit and water and to cut down on sugary drinks.'

© Guardian Newspapers Limited 2002

Fat . . . face the facts

Information from the Keep Fit Association

By Christine Gill, KFA Teacher & Community Dietitian, North Birmingham Community Trust

Minus points!

Deducted because:

Fats are fattening not filling. Weight for weight fat in foods provides more than twice the calories, 9 kilo-calories per gram compared to only 4 kilo-calories per gram for carbohydrate (starchy food) and protein. A modest 65gm chocolate bar with 11gms of fat contains the same calories as 6 large apples (with no fat). No prizes for guessing which would be the most filling! Could you eat 6 large apples as a snack and still find room for lunch?

Saturated fats (the type found in dairy products, meat products and some processed fat) are harmful as they raise the levels of cholesterol in the blood and increase the tendency of the blood to form clots. This can increase the risk of developing heart disease and stroke; therefore foods containing saturated fats should be taken in moderation.

Cancer risk is higher in countries with a high dietary fat intake. A high fibre intake from whole grain foods can be protective against cancer. Recent analysis of 40 studies implied that eating more than four servings a week of whole grain foods can reduce the risk by as much as 40% for many cancers.

Rates of obesity and overweight (often associated with high fat intake) have been steadily increasing in the UK for both adults and children. This increases risks for developing high blood pressure, diabetes, gallstones, osteoarthritis and heart disease in later life. Regular exercise reduces these risks.

Despite the recommendation for the population to reduce total fat intake to 35% of the total calories, records show that over the last 50 years it has been rising and is now around 40%. At the same time carbohydrate (starchy food) has decreased from 50% of the total calories to 45%. We need to reverse these trends to get the balance right.

Plus points!

Added because:

Essential fatty acids are just that – essential. Without them growth, brain function and the health of the skin may suffer. Foods such as vegetable oils and margarine (sunflower, corn, and rape-seed) and oily fish provide them.

Dietary fat helps us to absorb and can be a source of vitamins A, D, E and K which are needed for strong bones, night vision, healing and repair as well as maintaining good health.

Eating oily fish such as mackerel, herring, sardines, trout, salmon and pilchards has health benefits. They have been shown to reduce the tendency of the blood to clot. A study of Welsh men who had one heart attack but then ate two portions of oily fish each week showed that they reduced their risk of suffering a second attack by 30%.

Body fat acts as padding to protect vulnerable organs in the body such as the kidneys. Fat also serves as a fuel reserve when we are ill or have limited food available. One kilogram of body fat contains 7,000 kilo-calories of energy.

In women body fat influences fertility. A healthy woman will have between 18-25% of her weight as fat (12-15% for men). If body fat falls below around 15% for women periods will cease due to reduced oestrogen production.

How much?

Daily Guideline Intakes – These are based on average weight men and women with an average level of physical activity:

	Women	Men
Total Fat	70gms	95gms
Saturated Fat	20gms	30gms
Kcals	2000	2500

Food labels

These need understanding, values are given in 100gms. As a general guide:

- a lot is 20gms of fat per 100gms
- a little is 3gms of fat per 100gms

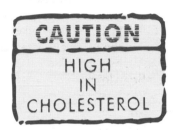

Getting the balance right

A balanced diet is based on starchy foods (bread, potatoes, rice, pasta) as these are filling not fattening and provide available energy for exercise. Enjoy eating at least five portions of fruit/vegetables daily. Using the plate model, two-thirds should come from starchy foods plus fruit and vegetables. A quarter is from dairy products (low fat milk, yoghurts, and cheese) together with lean meats and alternatives (fish, eggs, and beans). The smallest section shows that a modest intake of fatty/sugary foods is acceptable.

It is not just what you eat that matters, it is how much, how you cook it and how often you eat it. A little bit of what you fancy can do you some good!

- The above information is from the Keep Fit Association's web site which can be found at www.keepfit.org.uk

© *Keep Fit Association*

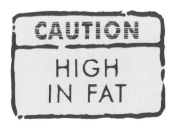

Confessions of a fitness fanatic

Eating less and exercising are simple cures for obesity but an addiction to activity can be just as unhealthy

By Matt Seaton

Fat is the new cancer. Last week, a conference on obesity warned that the government is not putting nearly enough resources into making us thinner, and that being overweight will soon rival smoking and drinking as the biggest drain on the nation's health services. The week before, we were told that obesity is reaching such epidemic levels among children that many can expect to be outlived by their less corpulent parents. Fat is a public menace, goes the message, and we're all going to hell – only not in a handcart, something more akin to a skip lorry, perhaps.

The answer? Simple: we should eat less and exercise more.

Exercise has tremendous benefits. It helps beat stress. It means you sleep better. It wards off depression. It gives you a sense of well-being – including, let's be honest, a sense of superiority over your less toned colleagues. It's an all-round panacea; so, yes, most of us should exercise more. But not me.

Don't get me wrong: I do exercise; I love exercising. The problem is, I love it too much. Obesity is not even a theoretical threat for me. The only way, frankly, I could ever weigh more than 13 stone would be if I swapped my obsessions with cycling and swimming for one with bodybuilding and started swallowing gallons of disgusting looking protein drinks. It's not likely, but I know the mentality.

Since it seems we're going to be hearing more about the exercise imperative, it's worth visiting what one might call the 'dark side' of fitness: the twilight world of the exercise addict. Take, for example, this sample week from the diary of one workout junkie I know:

Saturday: left house at 7am to fit in a two-hour bike ride.

Sunday: nothing – withdrawal symptoms noted, combined with wishful thoughts of attending swimming club training session.

Monday: swimming at lunchtime – good workout.

Tuesday: wanted to swim again in lunch hour, but was persuaded to play tennis instead. Slight feelings of regret (tennis not aerobic enough).

> *Exercise has tremendous benefits. It helps beat stress. It means you sleep better. It wards off depression. It gives you a sense of well-being*

Wednesday: took afternoon off work for long bike ride.

Thursday: met an old friend for a drink – but only after both have attended a swimming club session.

Friday: a day off, but only because another strenuous bike ride is scheduled for Saturday morning.

What we're looking at here is a clinical condition. This person feels sullied by inactivity after a single day; after two days, he is practically climbing walls.

Sustained deprivation from exercising leads first to irritability and restlessness, and then to determined and devious attempts to feed his habit. Finally, the subject's anxiety about his declining fitness leads to a near-psychotic state where he fantasises constantly about exercising.

You think I'm kidding? The diary, of course, was mine. Like all addicts, I think I have my problem 'under control'. In a healthier period,

MONDAY	WORK	LUNCH SWIM	WORK
TUESDAY	WORK	LUNCH SWIM TENNIS	WORK
WEDNESDAY	WORK	LUNCH	BIKE RIDE
THURSDAY	WORK	LUNCH	SWIM CLUB DRINKS
FRIDAY	///		BIG RIDE SAT
SATURDAY	7 A.M. 2 HR BIKE RIDE		
SUNDAY	NOTHING!		

I actually wrote a book about giving up cycling. Now I've relapsed, falling not so much off the wagon as back on to the bike.

Still, I believe my exercising can be 'managed'. Like an alcoholic who chews mints and hides bottles, I take great pains to present a veneer of normality. And I comfort myself that I'm nothing like as bad as some of the people I've seen in cycling and swimming clubs. The triathletes, for example, who make my own exercise compulsion look like a gentle stroll in the park.

A *New Yorker* article I once read about a woman who swam the Bering Strait (between Alaska and Siberia) quoted a statistic that eight out of 10 marathon swimmers suffer from some form of psychological stress. Not everyone deals with unhappiness by swimming the Channel (and neither does everyone who swims the Channel do so because they are dealing with unhappiness). It's a spectrum thing, though, and I do know people who suddenly found themselves going to the gym with a born-again zeal when a relationship broke up or a close relative died. Where some people hit the bottle, overeat or self-harm, the exercise addict works out.

There are more obviously destructive forms of dependency. Exercise does not, for instance, cause street crime. At least, I've never heard of anyone funding their gym subscription through mugging or burglary. What is more, exercise addicts are usually so full of endorphins they rarely need a prescription for Prozac.

Yet it does have costs. Exercise addicts conduct secret lives in which they furtively plan how they are going to score their next hit. Their need to work out interferes with their work, and deprives their families of their time. Such obsessional behaviour absorbs energy that might otherwise be deployed in more creative, less narcissistic ways. In short, excessive exercising makes one a very boring person indeed.

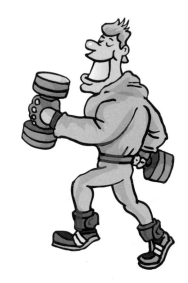

I sometimes cycle past people sitting outside a country pub, with pints in front of them, and think, 'That looks nice.' Those people might not be very fit, they might even be obese, but they're having fun. They have, in other words, what is commonly called 'a life'.

© *Guardian Newspapers Limited 2002*

Yes, the fittest do live longer . . .

. . . even fat smokers

The adage about the survival of the fittest is true, research reveals. An American study has found that people who exercise will live longer than those who do not, even if they smoke and are overweight.

The ten-year research on 6,000 middle-aged men was published in the *New England Journal of Medicine*. It found that the least fit were four-and-a-half times more likely to die within six years of the start of the study than were the most fit.

This was true whether or not the men had heart problems, smoked or were overweight.

A team at Stanford University, California, tested the men's fitness by monitoring them while they ran on a treadmill – usually used to check out the condition of the heart. Over time, the researchers found that the men's chances of staying alive rose significantly as their fitness increased.

'You are better off being fat and fit than skinny and sedentary,' said Dr Ken Cooper, a fitness expert.

'And you are better off smoking a pack a day and exercising regularly than being a non-smoker and sedentary.' The study found there was no need to exercise heavily, because going for a walk every day made a big difference to health. Dr Mike Stroud, Arctic explorer and author of *Survival of the Fittest*, said the results could be explained by evolution.

'Because of where we came from in evolution, we are meant to be active. Our whole biology is designed for activity,' he said.

'Therefore if you do not exercise you are more likely to run into trouble. People eat less then they used to and suffer from vitamin deficiency as a result, but it is not apparent because people do far too little exercise.

'Those vitamins contribute to the overall health of lungs, heart, bones and everything else.

'It is symptomatic of a society where everyone has cars and we all have a washing machine instead of a mangle.'

He said doing the gardening can be just as beneficial as going to the gym.

© *The Daily Mail, March 2002*

- The British Heart Foundation recommends 30 minutes of 'proper' exercise five times a week – including swimming, netball, football, tennis and rounders. (p. 1)

- Britain has the fastest growing obesity rate in Europe. (p. 1)

- On any given day, nearly 20% of Britons do no physical activity that lasts longer than 5 consecutive minutes. (p. 2)

- Some studies show that children who are more physically active showed higher academic performance. Team games and play promote positive social integration and facilitate the development of social skills in young children. (p. 3)

- Physical activity levels are low in the UK: only 37% of men and 25% of women meet the current guidelines (30 minutes' moderate activity on five or more days a week) suggested by the Government. (p. 4)

- Rates of serious weight problems have risen dramatically over the past decade, with nearly a third of children aged 16 classified overweight, and 17 per cent of 15-year-olds obese. (p. 6)

- In the US, 61% of adults are overweight. The average width of cinema and stadium seats has been increased from 17 inches to 22 inches. (p. 7)

- Only 5% of youngsters use their cycles as a form of transport in Britain as compared to 60-70% in Holland, and 30-40% of children are now taken to school by car, compared to 9% in 1971. (p. 8)

- A recent review showed that the average sustained weight loss over a minimum of 6 months was 4.0kg in 4 diet-only programmes, 4.9kg in 5 exercise-only programmes, and 7.2kg in 3 diet and exercise programmes. (p. 9)

- Recent studies have shown that children around the world are becoming increasingly sedentary – especially in poor urban areas. Time and resources devoted to physical education are being cut and computer games and television are replacing physically active pastimes. (p. 10)

- Preliminary data from a WHO study on risk factors suggest that inactivity, or sedentary lifestyle, is one of the 10 leading global causes of death and disability. (p. 11)

- In affluent nations obesity has been the fastest growing health epidemic for the past two decades. Many nations now record over 20% of their adult population as clinically obese and well over half the population as overweight. (p. 12)

- The lifestyle of couch potatoes has overtaken smoking as the major cause of ill-health in EU countries for the first time, the World Health Organization says. (p. 13)

- In Britain the proportion who are overweight or obese will increase from 48% last year to 52% in 2006. In France it will rise from 37% to 50%. (p. 17)

- Cardiovascular training includes anything that works your heart and lungs hard, such as brisk walking, jogging, swimming and cycling. Resistance training includes the use of weights and machines. (p. 20)

- Regular exercise, along with other things that make up a healthy lifestyle, can prevent some diseases that occur later in life and lead to a longer, happier life in general. (p. 21)

- It's recommended that teens do some sort of aerobic exercise at least three times a week, for 20 to 30 minutes at a time. (p. 21)

- Regular physical activity benefits communities and economies in terms of reduced healthcare costs, increased productivity, better performing schools, lower worker absenteeism and turnover, increased productivity and increased participation in sports and recreational activities. (p. 26)

- Exercise keeps your joints mobile and increases your circulation which makes your skin look healthier and you look younger. Above all it produces a wonderful feeling of well-being which makes you better able to deal with whatever life throws at you! (p. 27)

- The body is held together by a network of tissues and more than 600 muscles. Weakened muscles cannot support a heavy skeleton and so your posture will ultimately suffer. (p. 28)

- In order to lose weight it is essential to decrease energy intake below an individual's energy needs. In this way the additional energy which is needed by the body is taken from the existing body fat stores. (p. 31)

- Eating at the wrong times, and skipping meals altogether, leads to low blood sugar levels (hypoglycaemia). This results in tiredness, irritability, a lack of co-ordination, headaches, and a sudden urge to eat half a pound of chocolate! (p. 33)

- Despite the recommendation for the population to reduce total fat intake to 35% of the total calories, records show that over the last 50 years it has been rising and is now around 40%. (p. 37)

- The adage about the survival of the fittest is true, research reveals. An American study has found that people who exercise will live longer than those who do not, even if they smoke and are overweight. (p. 39)

ADDITIONAL RESOURCES

You might like to contact the following organisations for further information. Due to the increasing cost of postage, many organisations cannot respond to enquiries unless they receive a stamped, addressed envelope.

Association for the Study of Obesity (ASO)
20 Brook Meadow Close
Woodford Green
Essex, IG8 9NR
Tel: 020 8503 2042
Fax: 020 8503 2442
Web site: www.aso.org.uk
The ASO promotes research into the causes, prevention and treatment of obesity . . . encourages action to reduce the prevalence of obesity . . . and facilitates contact between individuals and organisations interested in obesity. Established the Obesity Resource and Information Centre (ORIC).

British Dietetic Association
5th Floor, Charles House
148/9 Great Charles Street
Queensway, Birmingham, B3 3HT
Tel: 0121 200 8080
Fax: 0121 200 8081
E-mail: info@bda.uk.com
Web site: www.bda.uk.com
The British Dietetic Association was formed to provide training and facilities for State Registered Dietitians. Today the Association has developed into a Professional Association. Runs the Weight Wise campaign.

British Heart Foundation (BHF)
14 Fitzhardinge Street
London, W1H 4DH
Tel: 020 7935 0185
Fax: 020 7486 5820
Web site: www.bhf.org.uk
The aim of the BHF is to play a leading role in the fight against heart disease and prevent death by ways including educating the public and health professionals about heart disease, its prevention and treament.

The Coronary Prevention Group
2 Taviton Street
London, WC1H 0BT
Tel: 020 7927 2125
Fax: 020 7927 2127
E-mail: cpg@lshtm.ac.uk
Web site: www.healthnet.org.uk

Contributes to the prevention of coronary heart disease, the UK's major cause of death. Provides information to the public on all preventable risk factors – smoking, high blood pressure and raised blood cholesterol and advice on healthy eating, exercise and stress. Produces publications.

European Food Information Council (EUFIC)
1 Place des Pyramides 75001
Paris, France
Tel: + 33 140 20 44 40
Fax: + 33 140 20 44 41
E-mail: eufic@eufic.org
Web site: www.eufic.org
EUFIC is a non-profit making organisation based in Paris. It has been established to provide science-based information on foods and food-related topics i.e. nutrition and health, food safety and quality and biotechnology in food for the attention of European consumers. It publishes regular newsletters, leaflets, reviews, case studies and other background information on food issues.

Fitness Industry Association
115 Eastbourne Mews
Paddington, London, W2 6LQ
Tel: 020 7298 6730
Fax: 020 7298 6731
E-mail: enquiries@fia.org.uk
Web site: www.fia.org.uk
The Fitness Industry Association is a non-profit trade association representing the entire health and fitness sector.

The Fitness League
52 London Street
Chertsey, Surrey, KT16 8AJ
Tel: 01932 564 567
Fax: 01932 567 566
E-mail: tfl@thefitnessleague.com
Web site: www.thefitnessleague.com
The Fitness League, a well-established nationwide exercise network, sponsored by Sport England and Sport Scotland, teaches rhythmic exercise to music. The TFL Technique is based on encouraging correct posture which releases the body's potential for good health

Institute of Food Research (IFR)
Norwich Research Park
Colney, Norwich, NR4 7UA
Tel: 01603 255000
Fax: 01603 507723
Web site: www.ifrn.ac.uk
The Institute of Food Research is a UK centre for research of international quality, sponsored by the Biotechnology and Biological Sciences Research Council. Their mission is to carry out independent basic, and strategic research on food safety, quality, nutrition and health.

Keep Fit Association
Suite 105, Astra House
Arklow Road
London, SE14 6EB
Tel: 020 8692 9566
Fax: 020 8692 8383
E-mail: kfa@keepfit.org.uk
Web site: www.keepfit.org.uk
The Keep Fit Association (KFA) gives thousands of us the opportunity to get together in a spirit of fun and friendship to exercise regularly together. Through our classes, we have successfully changed the lives of so many people by introducing them to fitness through movement and dance, resulting in more energetic, healthier and happier people all round.

World Health Organization (WHO)
20 Avenue Appia
1211-Geneva 27, Switzerland
Tel: + 41 22 791 2111
Fax: + 41 22 791 3111
E-mail: info@who.ch
Web site: www.who.ch
WHO works to make a difference in the lives of the world's people by enhancing both life expectancy and health expectancy.

INDEX

ACKNOWLEDGEMENTS

The publisher is grateful for permission to reproduce the following material.

While every care has been taken to trace and acknowledge copyright, the publisher tenders its apology for any accidental infringement or where copyright has proved untraceable. The publisher would be pleased to come to a suitable arrangement in any such case with the rightful owner.

Chapter One: How Fit Are We?

Overweight pupils 'doing hardly any exercise', © The Daily Mail, September 2002, *Plucky pensioners outpace teens*, © University of Essex 2002, *Physical activity and youth*, © World Health Organization (WHO), *Physical activity and coronary heart disease*, © British Heart Foundation, *Premature deaths from circulatory diseases*, © Crown copyright is reproduced with the permission of Her Majesty's Stationery Office, *Obesity linked to TVs in toddlers' bedrooms*, © Guardian Newspapers Limited 2002, *Obese children*, © The Daily Mail, September 2002, *Hungry for change*, © Guardian Newspapers Limited 2002, *Physical activity and obesity*, © The Obesity Resource and Information Centre (ORIC), *Think-tank calls for unhealthy food tax*, © Telegraph Group Limited, London 2002, *Myths about physical activity*, © World Health Organization (WHO), *Fears for 'generation of couch potatoes'*, © Telegraph Group Limited, London 2002, *The obesity pandemic*, © Andrew Prentice, London School of Hygiene and Tropical Medicine, *Couch potato lifestyle*, © Telegraph Group Limited, London 2002, *Jonah Lomu is fat . . .*, © Guardian Newspapers Limited 2002, *Wise up to your waist size*, © British Dietetic Association, *Britons stand tall, if slightly heavy in Europe*, © Guardian Newspapers Limited 2002, *Diet industry*, © Guardian Newspapers Limited 2002, *Nutrition news*, © EUFIC 2002.

Chapter Two: Physical Exercise

The benefits of exercise, © Absolute Fitness, *Be weight wise – be active*, © British Dietetic Association, *Why exercise is wise*, © KidsHealth, *Physical activity in children*, © British Heart Foundation, *Exercise and your heart*, © The Coronary Prevention Group, *Modes of travel to school*, © British Heart Foundation, *Physical activity*, © Crown copyright is reproduced with the permission of Her Majesty's Stationery Office, *Fitness at college*, © TheSite.org, *Personal trainer*, © TheSite.org, *Fitness the easy(er) way*, © TheSite.org, *The health benefits*, © World Health Organization (WHO), *A guide to healthy socialising and exercise*, © The Fitness League, *Exercise your way to a long and healthy life*, © Fitness Industry Association, *What is a healthy diet?*, © The Obesity Resource and Information Centre (ORIC), *The decreasing quality of children's diets*, © British Heart Foundation, *Food fitness*, © The Food and Drink Federation, *Sensible eating*, © Absolute Fitness, *Guidelines for a healthier diet*, © Institute of Food Research, *Obesity in children is increasing*, © British Heart Foundation, *Have a banana*, © Guardian Newspapers Limited 2002, *Fat . . . face the facts*, © Keep Fit Association, *Confessions of a fitness fanatic*, © Guardian Newspapers Limited 2002, *Yes, the fittest do live longer . . .* , © The Daily Mail, March 2002.

Photographs and illustrations:

Pages 1, 16, 24: Pumpkin House; pages 3, 8, 10, 13, 19, 23, 25, 28, 32, 36: Simon Kneebone; pages 6, 14, 27, 38: Bev Aisbett.

Craig Donnellan
Cambridge
January, 2003